Praise for *Pussy*

*"Talk about a tour de force! I am transfixed by the depth, humor,
and game-changing wisdom in this book. Regena is one of the most
profound and provocative thought leaders in the world today . . . and
she will wrestle a woman to the ground if need be to get her to give
up her resistance to her own desires and her pleasure. My charge to
you—as a doctor who has spent a lifetime assisting women
in healing their bodies—is that you have the courage to read*
Pussy: A Reclamation. *But don't just read it. Let the truth of it
sink into your body, right into your bone marrow. Let this book
change your life in the way it has changed mine."*

— from the foreword by **Christiane Northrup, M.D.**,
New York Times best-selling author of *Goddesses Never Age*

*"For years Regena Thomashauer has devoted herself to women, to
awakening their sensuality and their life force. This book is
the guide, the provocation, the initiation, the insistence,
the call to reconnect with the most vital, holy force in the world,
your pussy. It's time now! Read this and fly."*

— **Eve Ensler**, Tony Award–winning playwright, performer,
and activist; author of *The Vagina Monologues* and
In the Body of the World

*"Ladies, you are about to pledge allegiance to your greatest power.
Deeply positive and irresistible, Regena Thomashauer's work is
fueling a revolution of pleasure. This book is a total turn-on."*

— **Danielle LaPorte**, author of *The Desire Map*

PUSSY

PUSSY

A RECLAMATION

REGENA THOMASHAUER

HAY HOUSE, INC.

Carlsbad, California • New York City

London • Sydney • Johannesburg

Vancouver • New Delhi

The Library of Congress has cataloged the earlier edition as follows:

Names: Thomashauer, Regena, author.
Title: Pussy : a reclamation / Regena Thomashauer.
Description: 1st Edition. | Carlsbad, Callirfornia : Hay House, Inc., 2016.
Identifiers: LCCN 2016020272 | ISBN 9781401950248 (hardback)
Subjects: LCSH: Self-actualization (Psychology) | Motivation (Psychology) |
    Women--Psychology. | BISAC: SELF-HELP / Personal Growth / General. |
    SELF-HELP / Motivational & Inspirational. | HEALTH & FITNESS / Women's
    Health.
Classification: LCC BF637.S4 T484 2016 | DDC 155.3/339--dc23 LC record avail-
able at https://lccn.loc.gov/2016020272

Tradepaper ISBN: 978-1-4019-5026-2

10 9 8 7 6 5
1st edition, September 2016
2nd edition, April 2018

Printed in the United States of America

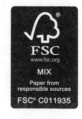
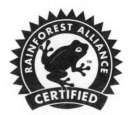

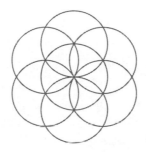

*I dedicate this book to the women
who will never hear of it, never even imagine it;
women who are currently living in the darkest
corners of the world (whether inner or outer),
who cannot even dream of having the luxury
to investigate the topics examined in the pages
that follow. Like the butterfly effect,
may these women somehow feel the impact
of our love and devotion to all things woman.
Even from afar, may our radiant light ignite theirs.*

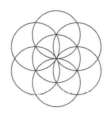

CONTENTS

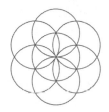

FOREWORD

Talk about a tour de force! I am transfixed by the depth, humor, and game-changing wisdom in this book. And honored to be the wingwoman in helping it soar all over Planet Earth. I can feel the trajectory of Regena's whole life and her soul's journey singing through every page, with the power to uplift the planet and every creature on it.

Regena is one of the most profound and provocative thought leaders in the world today. It is my hope that this book will put her work in the hands of every woman in this world so that they, like me, can know the life-changing information and practices revealed here.

My own initiation into the magic and mystery of the School of Womanly Arts began as the mother of two graduates. I got to see my daughters come to life and upgrade their relationships with themselves, with their friends, and with men. I have also been a frequent teacher at the school. Early on, I was lecturing on some aspect of women's wisdom and how it came through the body. Having spent a little time in the audience participating in some of the exercises, I began to make the connection between the experience of pleasure and rapture and its impact on physical health. And so, during a lecture, I asked the students to please come to the microphone and tell me if they had experienced any improvements in their physical health since starting the program at the SWA. I was astounded when the line of women at the microphone went to the back of the room. And then even more astounded as each woman related how her participation in the Womanly Arts had improved or healed everything from abnormal pap smears, infertility, and ovarian cysts to lung and breast cancer. It was then I knew that the deliberate pursuit of pleasure not only improved the quality of a woman's life—these things could also *save* her life.

There's plenty of science to support the pleasure/health connection. Part of the reason for this has to do with the production of massive amounts of a gas called nitric oxide, which is produced by the endothelial lining of the blood vessels during states of joy, pleasure, and ecstasy. And nitric oxide is the über-neurotransmitter that balances all the others—like dopamine, serotonin, and beta endorphin—the same neurotransmitters that so many women try to balance with psych meds like Prozac and Paxil, to name just two. I'm convinced that very few women would need these meds if they understood and applied the power of eros and pleasure in daily life.

Like a good mother, a good doctor, and a good scientist, I observed the life-giving power of pleasure in the lives of my daughters and other women. But then I realized that one doesn't reclaim the power of pussy with the intellect. This is a body trip. And as a woman, I too needed to dive into the SWA as a participant, not as some academic expert standing on the sidelines with a notebook in hand. And so—I dove in. I took the course. I became a full-fledged sister goddess. I learned how to brag, I learned how to praise other women. I learned the importance of having other sister goddesses in my life—women who no longer participated in the "mean girls" wounding so common in middle school, an artifact of Patriarchy from which the majority of adult women never recover unless they are open to being reeducated.

My daughters and I also worked through all kinds of mother-daughter chains of pain handed down from prior generations. They had to learn to see me as a sensual woman who desired a full, passionate life—not just a mother whose best years were behind her and whose future was limited to caring for grandchildren and other family members. I also sent scores of other women to the SWA, knowing that the key to women's health—and men's health and planetary health, for that matter—lay in reconnecting with this power source within us.

But there's more. I also experienced Regena's uncanny ability to intuit a woman's desires long before she herself is aware of them. In other words, Regena is a woman whisperer. And she will wrestle a woman to the ground if need be to get her to give up her resistance to her own desires and her pleasure. I've never seen anything like it. It's the best show in town. She is such a fearless warrior standing for sisterhood and pleasure. I was not immune.

Because of my work at the School of Womanly Arts, my whole life changed. At Regena's suggestion, I took up tango. I was both delighted and terrified, especially when she asked me to perform tango as an entrance for the Men's Session of Mastery, in front of hundreds and hundreds of men and women. The very same delight and terror that you may have felt when you first saw this book on the shelf or chose to pick it up in your hands. Regena had thrown down the gauntlet. Who was I to refuse the invitation? I danced not once, not twice, but three times. Each year taking it higher—and dancing better. Each year becoming more and more fearless in my willingness to sink into my body and into my pleasure. And each year attracting a more capable partner. Until finally I "landed it" when my tango teacher Paul agreed to go with me. And I trusted him completely. Just before we took the stage, Paul said, "I've got you." I melted into his arms and danced my heart out. And have been dancing regularly ever since. With every part of myself. Including my pussy.

Regena's work has also deepened my own work. It was a critical part of inspiring my most recent *New York Times* bestseller, *Goddesses Never Age*.

Because, as Regena says, reclaiming pussy is not about having sex with a lot of people. Nor is it about sex at all. Though it can be. Reclaiming pussy is about reclaiming the erotic power that is your Source as a woman. It's about bringing heaven down to earth—in the most sacred part of your body and your life. I've often said that if you want to know where your true power lies, go to those places you've been taught to fear the most. Your orgasm, your period, labor and birth, menopause—all processes that involve your pussy. This is where your real power lies. In the sacred temple of your pelvis. Right in front of the bone known as the sacrum—the holy bone. The place where the soul enters the body.

And so my charge to all of you—as a doctor who has spent a lifetime assisting women in healing their bodies—is that you have the courage to read *Pussy: A Reclamation*. But don't just read it. Let the truth of it sink into your body, right into your bone marrow. Let this book change your life in the way it has changed mine. Live the message. May you reclaim your radiance, wonder, and the life-giving power of pleasure and eros right in your own body. And thus remember who you really are. A goddess.

Christiane Northrup, M.D.
March 2016

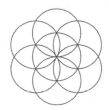

INTRODUCTION

Pussy.

It's arguably the most powerful pejorative word in the English language. It is the ultimate salacious smack to a woman's dignity, used when the intention is to hurt, humiliate, and fracture her humanity. *Pussy* is the lowest of the lows for men as well; there is no quicker way to snip a man's balls than to call him one, no clearer way to warn him that his reputation is in dire straits.

No one calls me "pussy" when they want to communicate how radiant and beautiful I look on a certain day. They don't use the word to tell me how expertly and thoroughly I have managed to accomplish a Herculean task. And yet, *pussy* is all that and more.

I am a woman of words, a gift I got from my father. He could jot a short line on a page and express everything he longed to say but lacked the social skill to impart. I grew up with him reading the Bible aloud, every Friday night. I was raised to have great respect and reverence for the power of language; for the way a simple, well-placed word could launch a movement or a philosophy. The way a single word could change the course of history.

My favorite book ever was the dictionary I received in junior high school. A cherished pastime was searching out the etymology of my favorite words, each turn of the page unpacking worlds of history. My problem? In all the millions of words I found between the covers of that beloved book, I could not find one single word that described *me*. No word that indicated my huge capacity to feel, my elusive and ever-changing cyclical nature, my raw femaleness, my delicacy, my shyness, my strength, my yearning to be seen and known and loved and gotten. No word. Not one.

We can learn just as much about a culture from what it's missing as from what it embraces.

One of the greatest pieces of unconscious conditioning we have in our Western culture is that we do not teach our children the name of the source of our feminine power. Ask my students at the School of Womanly Arts what they were taught to call their genitals as a child, and you'll get a parade of colloquialisms: Wickie, Cuckoo, Privates, Down There, Pooter, Pee Wee, the Fine China, Name and Address, Venus, Noonie, Miss Kitty, Purse . . . the list goes on. Those who were taught a more direct word were often taught to call it "vagina," a clinical term that is also physiologically incorrect.

But what's worse, the majority of women were taught to call it nothing at all.

When we have no common language to describe that which is most essentially feminine about us, we have no way to locate and own our power as women. As my dad used to read to us on Friday nights, "In the beginning was the Word." When there is no word, there is no beginning. How would you talk about an interconnected global computer network providing information and communication facilities via standard technological protocols if you did not have the word *Internet*? Yet our culture gives us no way to talk about the place where our power—and, in fact, all of life—comes from.

It's this very feminine power that is missing from all the success stories we hear. It's what leaves Sheryl Sandberg, one of the most productive women in America, revealing in a *New Yorker* profile that she's felt like a fraud all of her life. It's what has fashion designer Diane von Furstenberg admit on *CBS This Morning* that she wakes up every day feeling like a loser. It's what has Gayle King, who was interviewing von Furstenberg, reply that *she* wakes up every morning feeling fat.

It's what has Shonda Rhimes observe in her book, *Year of Yes*, that she and every other woman she knows push away compliments and are unable to receive appreciation and approval.

It's what has so many female grad students settling for assistant teaching, while their male counterparts head their own classrooms. (According to Linda Babcock, a professor of economics at Carnegie Mellon University and the co-author of *Women Don't Ask*, her very own dean explained the differential: "More men ask. The women just don't ask.") It's what has men initiate salary negotiations four times more often than women do. It's why when women *do* negotiate, they ask for 30 percent less than men.

I have been preoccupied with the question of why women have this limited ability to access their power and voice that nothing they do seems to ameliorate or resolve. As I look around the world of women, it seems as if our lights are off. *We* are turned off, like a light switch. The bulb is in there, but it sure isn't lit up. And it is no wonder. We have all been taught to turn off, to turn away.

Turn away from the homeless person begging for change. Turn away from the impact of climate change that we each deepen with our daily actions and inactions. Turn off from our own emotions.

No one had to teach us to turn off. Our culture models it with actions so much louder than words. So many of us were taught to back away from our strong emotions—to find them embarrassing, ridiculous even. So many of us were taught to keep a lid on anything and everything outrageous. To just turn it off. We turn off our life force, turn off our feelings, turn off our sensuality, and as a consequence, we turn off our power.

When we live in a world that cannot even comprehend its own inherent bigotry against women—and thus cannot step forward to honor or support the women and girls who have been devastated by it—what is the recourse? How do we stand up to an invisible assault that does not want to be made visible? How does a woman weather—let alone triumph over—such a global denial of her experience?

How does she locate a pathway to mend, strengthen, and remake herself in a world that does not recognize she is broken?

How does she turn on when she has been systematically denied, passed over, and subjugated?

Where is the opportunity in this story line for the victim to become the heroine?

How do we, as women, reconsecrate our holiness after we have been defiled, turned off, and ignored all our lives?

The solution for the epidemic of powerlessness among women, which neither great success nor higher education is able to solve, is simple: reconnecting a woman to her pussy. Just as pussy is the source of all human life, pussy is the source of each woman's connection to her own life force, her voice, and her sense of internal power. When a woman turns on her pussy, she is actually turning on her life force and connecting to her divinity.

My life's work has been about creating this very pathway for women: the missing pathway out of victimhood and into our own inherent radiance. A pathway that does not depend on anything or anyone, but rather places the power firmly in a woman's own hands. When she designs, and then lives, her own destiny, a woman naturally sets right everything wrong in our world. But the first step is the most crucial—she has to get right with her own pussy. More than right. She has to *turn on* the most disparaged, maligned, and unknown part of herself.

As the woman behind the School of Womanly Arts, a multi-million-dollar women's educational institution based in New York City, I have made it my mission and my purpose to reclaim our power—to reclaim *pussy*, starting with the very word. I do it through the courses I teach, where I usher hundreds of women through personal growth and transformation. I take women on a journey that includes historic reckoning, sensual awakening, psychological reconfiguration, and spiritual and physical reconnection. I immerse my students in the Womanly Tools and Arts, invite them into a sustainable community of thousands of sisters they can learn from and depend on, and extend their growth and transformation throughout the rest of their lives. The School of Womanly Arts (which I'll refer to throughout this book as the SWA) is created of women, by women, and for women. Its not-so-secret purpose is to initiate each student into full possession of her inalienable, indefatigable, and indestructible feminine spirit in the face of life's eternal, ongoing challenges. A woman who graduates from our programs takes with her a sense of connection to her irrevocable power, a depth of confidence previously unimaginable, and a righteous understanding of her value during this time and place on earth.

Picture this: a room filled with the crackling connected pulsing energy of hundreds of women, standing together in sisterhood, some for the first time, some as core community members for years, all instantly bonded. Every key of a woman's emotional, physical, and spiritual keyboard is invited to play. We rage madly together, weep to our ancient bones together, and raise the roof dancing in rapturous celebration of the privilege of life itself, together. Each woman feeling more *herself* because of the presence of the others.

And that is precisely what is going to happen for you in reading this book. You are going to connect more powerfully than you could have ever imagined to your deepest intuition, your sacred feminine power, and your voice that needs to be heard. I am going to give you some of the exercises that I use in the SWA's Mastery program, so you won't just read about what's possible, you will actually experience incredible changes inside yourself as you practice along with me.

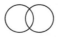

A DISCLAIMER

In this book, I am going to use the distinctions *man* and *woman* as a structure for talking about the masculine and feminine forces in the world.

I know and love all my readers—gay, straight, bi, transgender, and otherwise—and this book is for women of all orientations. Masculine and feminine energies are at work in all individuals, in all relationships, and in the world in general. The majority of us have been taught so much about our masculine energies, and very, very little about the feminine, resulting in a challenging imbalance both individually and collectively. This book will rebalance your inner scales.

Regardless of sexual preference or gender identity, we all have masculine and feminine within us. The feminine force is primarily responsible for desire. The masculine force is primarily responsible for the production of that desire. The masculine is the rock; the feminine is the wave crashing against that rock. In same-sex relationships, these roles are often swapped back and forth, but they are often swapped in hetero relationships as well. Sometimes a hetero woman will enjoy slipping into her masculine, and a hetero man will enjoy inhabiting his feminine.

I will do my best to pay tribute to all the different constructs as I write. And, for clarity, I will use *men* and *women* as reference points. My goal is to allow you to really crystallize the differences between masculine and feminine energies, regardless of which bodies they're showing up in. That way, all of us can begin to truly enjoy the polarity between—and the union of—these two forces in our world.

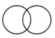

This book is my offering. It contains everything I have learned, everything I have longed to share with a wider audience than could possibly fit into the enormous ballrooms and theaters where I meet my students each year. It will walk you through the journey that each woman takes in the Mastery program, which mirrors the journey that each woman takes in her life.

The centerpiece of this protocol? You guessed it: a reclamation of the very source of her feminine power.

We begin with a reconciliation that is tragic in its very necessity. I reacquaint each student with that part of herself that is the key to everything she has ever been looking for but has been pushed into shadow, into shame. A part that has, for all intents and purposes, gone underground. Unnameable, undiscussable. Left to fend for itself or worse, to wither and die. And how else would I begin this reconciliation but in the way our very world began—with a word?

In the beginning was the Word.

The word, my darlings, is *pussy.*

And with this book, I intend to return that word to its rightful place—as the highest of all possible compliments, as a sacred living prayer.

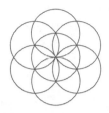

CHAPTER 1

THE CALL OF THE GODDESS

The valley spirit never dies,
It is named the Mysterious Feminine.
And the doorway of the Mysterious Feminine
Is the base from which heaven and earth sprang.
It is there within us all this while.
Draw upon it as you will, it never runs dry.

— TAO TE CHING

Every other summer or so, for the past 40 years, I have met up with my two best cousins for a girls' weekend. There's Hannah, who lives in Colorado with her husband, son, and daughter, and Grace, who lives in Houston with her husband and four girls.

Back when we were in high school in Philadelphia, we were three young women with very big dreams. Hannah was a sculptor, a poet, a painter. Grace was a very talented photographer who worked on the school newspaper. I was an actress.

We watched one another's lives unfold—witnessing, supporting, and loving one another to the best of our abilities.

Miraculously we stayed tethered as each of us moved in radically different directions, made different choices, and created different lives for ourselves and our children.

Hannah had dated all the wrong men, often investing her money to make their dreams come true. She dabbled in pottery, dabbled in porcelain, and dabbled in running an art studio. She was a brilliant potter but was never able to charge quite what she was worth for her work, as she never really felt worthy. Finally she met a great guy, a director and owner of a wilderness program, married him, and had kids. They raised the kids outdoors, camping in the summer, skiing all winter, and growing their own organic food.

Grace went in a different direction. She married a wealthy trust-fund boy whose family was in oil, and gave up her dream of being a photojournalist while she had four children. She volunteered a few hours a week at the Houston Children's Charity, and served on the PTA. Her marriage was old-school: She gave all the decision-making over to her husband. They lived where he wanted to live, went to the church he preferred every Sunday (even though she hated it), and joined the country club where his family belonged. The full-time responsibility for raising the kids fell to her, as her husband was often away on business and social ventures with the long-standing members of his exclusive community. Sometimes she felt like she was just a broodmare, brought in to supply him with heirs.

These two beloved cousins of mine watched with curious and sometimes critical eyes as I created the School of Womanly Arts and wrote three books. They danced at my wedding, supported me through my divorce, and taught me what they knew about being a good mom. But they never set foot in my school. Taking a class at the SWA was way too weird, way too scary. Even my visits to their homes in the summers could be off-putting. One year I wanted to bring some fun on a visit to Hannah's. I brought a playlist and an iPod and had us all dance for no reason in the kitchen. After I got home, Hannah called and asked me to please not do that again because it upset the children. Moms, I took this to mean, were supposed to be serious—fun and turn-on were not on the menu.

I watched as both of these women put their radiance and joy on a *waaaay* back burner, in deference to raising kids and organizing households. But still I longed for my cousins to come experience my classes and to see what I had been creating all these years. I wanted to share all my discoveries with them; I wanted to see how my work might contribute to their lives and how it might support them in all the myriad responsibilities they had. It was so hard, they kept telling me, to make time to travel to New York, what with the kids and schedules and work. But I never stopped inviting them. Every time there was an upcoming class, I called and cajoled.

After about 10 years of asking, Hannah finally said yes.

My father had just died, and I needed to bring my mom to the course I was teaching that weekend. (There was no sitting shiva because of the High Holy Days.) Later, my mom would start to help me teach at the SWA. Now she is the "Bubbe"—the Grandmother or Elder—of the School. She assists me by taking aside any women who are having challenges with the material. She pulls them onto her lap, hears their stories of devastation, and dries their tears, then sends them back to class.

But all those years ago, I simply invited Mom to come to the School that weekend so she would not be alone. And I asked Hannah if she would come and sit next to Mom, supporting her for the weekend. Hannah said yes in a heartbeat. Interesting, isn't it, that she could find her way into the School of Womanly Arts classroom only when she was there on behalf of someone else? This is such a common thing for women in our culture. It's very difficult for us to say yes to our own pleasure. We have no experience prioritizing our own joy or making an investment in ourselves. But it is very easy to say yes to responsibility and obligation. We are highly motivated when we can be of service to someone else.

Still, you can't imagine the joy it brought me to have Hannah there! It was thrilling. And wouldn't you know it, Hannah fell in love with the SWA. So much so that she joined me in the campaign to get Grace to come the next semester, when she decided to do the full course herself.

Now I was living my dream: I had both my cousins in attendance! These were the women who had long inspired me with the sustaining power of loving friendship and all-night laughs; who had taught me to value and honor sisterhood. To some degree because of them, I had created a huge community of women to support and love one another at the School of Womanly Arts. And now I had the privilege of introducing them to the body of work that had inspired me and changed the trajectory of my life.

The School of Womanly Arts is an initiation into womanhood. Not the womanhood that's about servitude and service, but rather the ancient indigenous knowledge of who and what a woman is. About the inherent, unaccessed power that every woman possesses. Every aspect of *woman* is unpacked—sensuality, body, health, spirituality, career, self-worth, confidence. Most important, each student is taken through the transformation from girl to woman, where she has the opportunity to trade in her self-doubt, self-hatred, and self-deprecation for a deep-seated sense of her own power. She finds herself rooted in a community of support and love that allows her to fulfill her dreams and destiny in a way she could not have previously imagined.

Hannah and Grace took the class together. But what they did with the material afterward was quite different. Hannah jumped in with both hands and feet—and everything between. She brought her husband to a session for men, which he loved. She practiced the tools of the Womanly Arts in her life back home. She brought all her best friends from Denver to the School, to deepen her sense of community. Her sex life with her husband took off. Even after his brush with prostate cancer, she was able to apply what she had learned at the SWA and restore them to a happy, healthy sex life. She took a big financial risk and had them buy and renovate her dream house, which she designed and decorated. She enjoyed that so much, she found a space in town to rehab and create an arts center for her community, where she gives classes in pottery making. She hires other artists to hold classes in painting and drawing, and rents studio space to whoever needs it. The arts center has become her new passion. She even returned to graduate school to study business in order to learn how to best manage, and perhaps even scale, the arts center. She is rocking all of her classes. She has found her voice, her passion, her radiance. These days, dance breaks in her kitchen are common, and her kids roll their eyes in secret delight. She and her husband have never been happier.

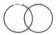

THE WOMANLY ARTS

Throughout this book, I will refer frequently to the Womanly Arts—the concepts at the heart of the work I do—and the tools that support them. These Tools and Arts were thoroughly described in my first book, *Mama Gena's School of Womanly Arts*. When a woman puts these concepts into practice in her life, her entire life will change. Many of them will be mentioned here, some will be covered in detail; you can also find them encapsulated in the appendix for a down-and-dirty review. These tools can be used on a daily basis to keep your orbit high and to keep you plugged into your divine power source. They are also super handy in an emergency, when you are suffering a temporary loss of sanity and you need to switch gears quickly and find your center.

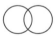

Grace's life, on the other hand, is very different. She did not continue practicing the Tools and Arts she learned in Mastery and she did not take advantage of the support of her fellow students— the ongoing community we call Sister Goddesses.[1] She and her hus-

---

[1] I call the participants in my courses, and the women who have read my books, "Sister Goddesses" to remind us that all women on this planet are sisters to one another, and all of us are divine. Treat a woman like a sister, and a goddess, and you bring out the best in her.

band have been hiding his excessive drinking for years, and their lives have continued to shrink to accommodate the constraints of his alcoholism. He's been carried out of the country club on too many occasions to name, and he was thrown off the board of the family business for reasons he never shared with Grace. All along, she has been doing her best to cover his tracks and hold the family together. He's told her he will divorce her and leave her with nothing if she tries to get him help for his addiction.

The secrets that Grace has been forced to keep have bled into the next generation. Her daughter has dropped out of college after failing all her classes because she was date-raped and never felt right enough about herself to report the crime or get counseling. She has moved back home in shame. When we were together for our last girls' weekend, Grace confessed that she has known, deep in her heart, that keeping her husband's—and now her daughter's—secrets has been wrong, but she hasn't had the gumption to speak her own truth.

Grace also confessed to me that she loved the SWA, but that her husband had complained a lot while she was enrolled. She had to travel to New York one weekend a month for four months and wasn't there to look after the family. Apparently he'd expected her to come home each weekend ready to have lots of sex with him. When it didn't happen that way, he didn't know what she was getting out of it. Grace had taken the class with her friend Shelley, who studies *A Course in Miracles* with her. Shelley told Grace after the second weekend that she did not believe all the talk about the importance of connecting to one's sensuality. The most important thing, she insisted, was to connect with your *heart*, not your pussy. Grace decided Shelley had a point. As much as she enjoyed the spectacle of the SWA, she decided she did not need the content. It was much easier to disapprove of something new, different, and confronting than it was to risk opening herself to a brand-new viewpoint.

So both of my dear friends got the call of the Goddess. The difference? Hannah picked up—while Grace let the call go through to voice mail.

Now you get that same choice. This book is meant to offer you everything I teach at the School of Womanly Arts Mastery program. All the concepts and material that I have developed and thoroughly tested to initiate you into the life you've always wanted and teach you how to sustain that life over time. This book is a culmination of 30 years of personal research and 20 years of running the School. It's the same program that has already transformed the lives of thousands of women, including my cousin Hannah.

And now it's your turn. My darling, the Goddess is calling. Are *you* ready to answer?

THE CALL OF THE GODDESS

I got the call early. From the time I was six years old, the Goddess would come visit me at night. She would sit on my bed, on that spot between the pillow and the bed's edge. I couldn't exactly see her, but I knew she was there, in the way a six-year-old just *knows*.

At first I was terrified. I would freeze, not move an eyelash, because I wanted her to think I was asleep. I wanted her to go away.

But over time, my fear of this nightly apparition melted. I started to relax into the experience of her. Her presence produced a feeling inside me that was unlike anything I had ever felt before. It was a sensation of weightless warmth, where my insides turned to liquid gold.

I would remain perfectly still, allowing her to seep into my consciousness. Taking her in. Feeling her perfect yearning. I remember the feeling of wanting to hold her, to inhabit her, to *know* her.

But there were no words between us, and I could not look at her. Each time I turned my head to look directly at her, she vanished.

No matter. She awakened love in me. Not love like you'd feel for a mother; love of the way she made me feel.

Sensuous love.

Sensual love.

And a profound, unmistakable holiness.

In her presence, I felt radiant.

It was a feeling I now recognize. It was *turn-on*.

Even though I was only six, the turn-on I felt was so deep; so utterly *me*. A feeling that spread all over my body and seeped into my cells, like a mountain of warm butter on a hot English muffin. This feeling was my earth, my spirit, my eternity, my here and now.

Simple, essential. Like sunshine. I knew it was the most precious feeling in the world.

I imagine you might know the feeling too.

If the smell of freshly baked bread were a feeling, it would be that. If the last warm day of fall were an emotion, it would be that.

The feeling of being utterly and completely present, besotted with the gift of life itself. Transported by the privilege of existence. No goal, just pure enjoyment. A sunset can create this inner ooze. Or the smell of your baby's head. Riding your horse. The ocean. Connection. Laughter. Ecstasy in any form.

That's what the Goddess felt like.

I could feel her silent yearning for me. She wanted to be known by me. She wanted to be seen, noticed, heard, felt. She wafted like perfume inside of me. I melted at her presence, enchanted. I would do anything to serve her. I felt safe. Found. Utterly myself. And in service to her, and this feeling in me, forever.

This experience lasted only a couple of years, but it has created a lasting effect on my life. My grown-up mind wonders, now, if these experiences with the Goddess were a dream or a fantasy. Perhaps they were a self-protective response to growing up in a household infused with patriarchal religious values, male-centric social customs, and physical abuse. The Goddess represented the exact opposite of these things; she became a kind of guardian angel in my life, as well as the subject of my ongoing philosophical quest. Everything I encountered in those years that was masculine and "spiritual" equated to pain and suffering. The Goddess encounters were the precise opposite; they were feminine, they were sacred, and they felt delicious.

At the time, *delicious* was not a word I associated with being a woman. I did not see any deliciousness, anywhere, when it came to being an adult female. What I saw in my mother's life—and in the lives of the other women in the neighborhood—was nothing I wanted for myself. I saw women who prioritized their husbands and families, who worked very hard, who shopped and cooked and cleaned and drove station wagons and made everyone else's lives run smoothly I saw women who were self-sacrificing, who ignored their own needs, who gave up on their own happiness. I saw women who were being subjugated. Women who were being undervalued at their jobs. I saw women who looked empty, hollow, and dead inside; women who were angry, bitter, resentful, resigned. I saw a world of women who lacked the fiery sense of life and liveliness that comes from living passionately and feeling deserving of goodness. I saw a world of women whose lights were dim, if not extinguished. The job description for "woman" was nothing I wanted to sign up for.

The experience of the Goddess was the first time I felt a different kind of beckoning. I felt a sense of promise, a sense of inspiration in womanhood that was unlike anything I was witnessing around me. It was an energetic essence of the feminine that I had not previously encountered. It had nothing to do with laundry or cooking dinner or servitude in any form.

Being with the Goddess was not about *doing* anything. It was simply about *experiencing her presence.* Every part of my skin felt enlivened. Something in me was awakened, as if a light switch in my soul had been turned on.

This was a huge deal for me. I had suffered the abuse of an older brother from the time I was an infant. When a child suffers physical and verbal abuse, her soul flies out of her body in self-protection. This experience robbed me of a sense of ease and safety and comfort, both in the world and in my body. But it was so much a part of my life and my sense of home that I did not clock it as a problem. (It wasn't until much later in my life that it finally stopped me in my tracks.) My story is by no means unique. Far too many women have experienced abuse and unchecked violence in this world, with no consequence to the abuser and no assistance for the victim. In the pages that follow, I offer you my story—in hopes it will assist you in finding your own. Mine is a teaching story. It is a story that is meant to inspire. To help you reframe your priorities and set you loose into a deeper, sweeter part of yourself. Into an experience of rightness, where you can stand before yourself and feel proud, powerful, moved. Grateful for every step that has made you and remade you into the woman you are today.

You. As heroine, as legend, every mundane day. May who I am awaken and inspire you to see who *you* are.

Because I am the definition of a powerful woman.

I love with my whole body, heart, and soul.

I say whatever the fuck is on my mind.

I make huge mistakes proudly.

I rage with as much passion as I grieve.

I live my poetry, my art.

I mother my child like a she-wolf.

I risk my life to live my truth.

I laugh easily, mostly at myself.

I would sell my soul for a night of ecstasy.

And every day I'm serving my Goddess, and my God, with every cell of my being.

In other words, I am just like you.

SPYING FOR THE GODDESS

Right around the time the Goddess started visiting me, I remember waking up one morning and walking over to the window of my pink bedroom. As I gazed outside, I realized—with a six-year-old's version of consternation—that I was no longer looking forward to the day. I knew myself as a person who looked forward to days, but that feeling was gone. What had replaced it was a feeling of deadness inside my body. The river of goodness that is our birthright had dried up inside of me.

And even though I was young, I knew something was wrong with a world that would take enthusiasm away from a child. A world that would make me feel worried and wrong. That would make me feel not good enough, simply because I wasn't born a boy. That would consign me to the experience of daily abuse, with no end in sight. I knew the feeling of goodness I'd learned from the Goddess was *truth*. I also knew that she was in some way counting on me to take a stand for that truth in the world. Over the years, she faded from my bedside. But I felt her inside of me and somehow knew she had awakened me to this path.

I vowed to set the problem right in my lifetime.

Nothing and no one could have removed me from this mission. I was looking for a feeling of rapture, the feeling I got in the presence of the Goddess. I wanted it all the time. And I could see that this feeling belonged to children but died as they grew into teenagers and adults. Everywhere. I sensed that this was human error and therefore correctable. And correction was necessary for all concerned.

I was looking for the feeling that I knew, in some unnameable way, was the locus of both my fragile humanness and my divinity. The intersection between me and that which was greater than me. The grace inherent in every moment, every person, every pebble, whose felt sense is an immeasurable enthusiasm for life itself.

I decided I had to figure out what had happened to my enthusiasm, and to that of so many children and grown-ups I knew. Not only figure it out, but *fix* it. I knew intuitively it would involve locating the Goddess and returning her to her rightful place. And, I figured, since she had come to me, it was *my* job to find her where she was hiding.

I started locally, hitting up the many synagogues in my neighborhood. I thought maybe the Goddess was reformed, and it was just that we were conservative. But no. No Goddess anywhere. In fact, you really couldn't find a more unrapturous place than the suburban synagogue of my youth.

Next I went interdenominational. I checked out the churches, hitting up the Catholics first, with my friend Susan O'Hara. Her mom looked at me suspiciously when I asked to attend Mass with the family. I thought maybe she suspected I was a spy, but she let me come anyway. I liked the fabulous gowns on the guys swinging the incense, and the decor was high and holy fancy. But, alas, no Goddess there either. Just dreary disapproval. No joy.

I thought I'd hit the jackpot when my family spent a summer in Israel. I was 14. It was a spying frenzy! I went to mosques and churches. The Mount of Olives, the Baha'i Temple, Mount Sinai, the Dome of the Rock, the Cave of Machpelah, Masada, the Church of the Holy Sepulchre, Via Dolorosa, the garden of Gethsemane, the Wailing Wall. All the while scribbling in my notebook, à la Harriet the Spy. But everything I saw was the same: old, dusty, empty of life, empty of joy, filled with angst and blind soulless compliance in the name of some vengeful kind of God. I was there to search for Her, but from my vantage point there was nothing holy about these places.

What's more, the so-called Holy Land proved dangerous for a young blonde girl with an open, searching spirit. I was molested almost everywhere I went. Leered at. Touched inappropriately. Demeaned. Violated. In the marketplace. On the street. And, devastatingly, at many holy shrines.

I did not know what this inappropriate attention was or how to stop it. I literally had no idea what was happening, I just knew it was wrong. I did not understand that my short dress, white skin, and blond hair announced, "Come molest me." In the public pool, at the hotel, on the bus. Anywhere I was unprotected. And no one else seemed to see or notice. Even though it was happening under everyone's noses, there were no words to talk about it. There were no words to talk about the transition between girl and young woman, no words to express being viewed as a provocative object—rather than the child I was—in a foreign culture. No words to justify the deep sense of wrongness I felt about myself. No words between my mother and me, between my father and me, between my brothers and me. So it was as if it wasn't happening.

Not surprisingly, my spying was going poorly. Very poorly. I wanted so much to find the Goddess, but she wasn't anywhere to be found in the Holy Land. I was confused. How could they call it "holy" if She wasn't anywhere in sight?

We were in Israel long enough for me to have a horrifying summer in which I learned to fear and distrust men and to curse my emerging womanhood. Long enough to awaken me further to the danger I was in, as a very old girl and a very young woman in this world.

I lost faith. Hung up my trench coat, put away my notebook, and became even more introverted, shy, and unhappy. I believed for certain that the Goddess was extinct, like a dodo bird or a Tyrannosaurus rex. She had been eliminated as a by-product of progress. I knew it was highly unlikely I would ever find her. I had very nearly given up.

Losing Her, Finding Her

I moved to New York City right after college. I did a bit of traveling for some regional theater, working at intervals with Shakespeare & Company and the Wyoming Shakespeare Festival, and taking acting classes. But in truth, my life was slowly grinding to a halt. I was an actress who was not acting, a singer who was not singing, a young woman who was not dating or developing socially. My confidence was shrinking. I was waiting tables and hiding from everyone whose expectations I was so conscious I was disappointing.

I had broken up with my wonderful college boyfriend—he just loved me too much. His love felt foreign to me. Since I had never experienced anything like it from my dad or brothers, it just felt wrong. I knew if I couldn't handle a relationship with a man this wonderful, there had to be something wrong with me. I was flooded with doubts. Was I gay? Unloving? Why couldn't I connect? And how could I stand on a stage with all these unanswered questions about myself as a woman?

So instead of accepting a job for another season at Shakespeare & Company, I went into therapy. After years on the couch, my self-doubt and self-hatred only grew worse, and I retreated more and more. I finally decided to quit therapy and study on my own. I dove into Greek and Roman mythology, archetypes, and the work of Carl Jung and Joseph Campbell; the ancient goddess traditions and indigenous cultures. I learned that in these early religions, it was the Great Mother—rather than just the Heavenly Father—who was worshipped. That throughout prehistoric and early historic periods of human development, entire *religions* existed in which people revered their supreme creator as female. And rather than an assumed division between spirit and matter, these cultures believed there was spirit *in* matter. Holiness was everywhere, not only in churches or temples. Death was just as revered as birth, and it was celebrated with joy and gratitude. The feminine was honored as the portal to life, and everything and everyone was holy.

It all made much more sense to me than the religions of my childhood. I was so hungry for my discoveries that I studied myself right into being a celibate hermit. I believed the things I was learning and discovering were so alien to the patriarchal world culture that I was a part of that no one would understand what I was talking about or what I was doing. These eternal verities only seemed to make me feel *more* disenfranchised from the world, because I was so certain that no one would share or empathize with my findings. I was cut off from my friends, my family, and the work I loved most. All in the name of healing myself and solving the riddle of my life.

Then, everything changed.

One of the waitresses I worked with invited me to a class she was taking at The Actors Information Project. One of the teachers came up to me after I'd done my audition piece. "Regena," he said, "you are a really good actress. But there is absolutely no sensuality in your work. If you don't find a way to connect with that part of you, you will continually be cast in roles much older than you are."

This comment shook me up. It also made good sense to me: I had not dated or had a lover in many years. I knew this was an area I had no skill or talent in; I had failed at my relationship with my amazing boyfriend, and I had no interest in failing again.

I still had so much fear of men.

But I also wanted to be an actress. My desire to live that dream was just barely greater than my fear.

Upon hearing my plight, another one of the acting teachers told me about a class he had recently taken at More University called Basic Sensuality. He said it would help me bring more sensuality to my work as an actor. The whole idea of this terrified me. It's safe to say I would rather have leapt out of a plane, gone deep-sea diving, or cleaned the streets with a toothbrush than take a class in sensuality.

I was so nervous in the week or so leading up to the class. I kept trying to think of reasons not to attend. I was a bit like Boo Radley; I had not been out of the house much in the previous eight years. It had taken a lot for me to go to that acting class in the first place. Now I was being encouraged to dive into the part of myself I feared the most—the part of me that had experienced so much abuse. I had no way of connecting to my sensuality—except through repulsion.

But something greater than me drew me forward.

The class was held in a brownstone on the Upper West Side of Manhattan. I immediately hated it. I had never seen stranger, more abhorrent people than the participants, and the teachers were a bunch of unattractive, aging hippies. I felt so out of place, so disconnected, that I could barely stay in my seat. I wanted to run home and hide. Instead I sat in the last row, not speaking to anyone. When it was time for the lunch break, I did run home, intending to stay there, where it was safe. But something forced me back for the afternoon session. (That, I would soon learn, is the magnificent power of desire: it presses you forward even when your mind is screaming, *"Stop!!"*)

The topic of the class was how our culture restricts us from experiencing pleasure. The teachers spoke about how everyone is perfect, yet none of us feels that way because our culture teaches us to hate and criticize ourselves. They had us examine what they called our "stable data"—the unspoken messages of limitation and criticism we received in childhood. Then they described the many ways to experience, and to give, sensual pleasure. This was all new to me, and very shocking, and kind of horrible, and only a very teeny-tiny bit wonderful.

At day's end, we got a homework assignment. We were to prepare our home as if the most important person in the world were coming to visit us. How would we entertain them? Would we clean the house? Purchase special foods, candles, flowers, music? What would we wear? The trick of the homework was that *we* were the guests: all the preparations were for ourselves. Why? Well, most people only set out the candles and fine china for company. This was a chance to treat ourselves in a special way.

Once our senses were pampered, we were to disrobe and look at ourselves in the mirror. We were to observe what we liked about ourselves, and then touch ourselves for sensual pleasure. To me, this assignment sounded utterly foolish and completely nerve-wracking at the same time. But I had always been a good student, so I decided to do it to the best of my ability. I had never created a special night of pleasure just for myself. I had created nice things for other people, but never just for me.

I left the class and stopped at the corner deli in my neighborhood to pick up some treats. I had been anonymously visiting this market for many years. No one had ever noticed me. Tonight was different. I didn't understand what was happening, but as I walked around the market it was as if little sparks of attraction were flying off my skin. I noticed that instead of being invisible, as I usually was, I was being noticed by the men who worked at the shop. It seemed everyone wanted to help me! I was not used to being sought after or seen, so it was scary and wonderful. I was enjoying their attention, but it felt overwhelming to me at the same time.

I bought myself pink roses, Pellegrino, dark chocolate with almonds, French bread, Gruyère cheese, and strawberries. Then I scurried home with my little bundle of things and cleaned up my apartment as if someone special were arriving. I cleaned the bathtub, put all the laundry away, vacuumed, and did the dishes.

Then I set out a beautiful platter and arranged all my goodies. I put some Sade on the stereo and took a long, delicious bath with the music playing, my little tray of treats spread out by the tub.

And I noticed something. Time . . . altered. Instead of being a rushing river trouncing and bouncing me, time became a calm lake, of which I was the mistress. It felt like it was my experience of pleasure that controlled time. *I* was in control. I was in *control.* There was an actual *physical consequence* to this experience of taking my pleasure. It had started in the outside world, as the guys in the grocery store started to magnetize toward me. And now I was doing something that I had never, ever done: creating a small, exquisite celebration for myself. For me. Only me. With only my pleasure in mind.

And then it happened. The *Goddess* feeling.

That melt-my-insides, liquid-golden-honey-pouring-inside-and-out feeling. Utter relaxation. Utter surrender. Utter attunement to the most beautiful-powerful-grateful part of me. A universal feeling of connection.

A feeling I hadn't had since childhood.

Dazed and amazed, I stepped out of the tub and proceeded to the next stage of the assignment. I was to look at myself in the mirror, lit by candles, and notice what was beautiful. I had never thought to look at myself like this, to notice my own beauty. I had only ever looked in the mirror to criticize myself—to see if I was too fat, or having a bad hair day, or if I had a pimple. To my utter surprise, when I looked for my beauty, I was completely enraptured with my reflection. I found myself to be so radiant, so lovely, and so touchingly gorgeous. I used a hand mirror and looked at my back. I am not sure I had ever seen my back before. It was strong and well-shaped. The curve of my spine was so elegant. I felt deeply moved that, in all the years of having these shoulders, this spine, this back, I had never noticed how it was a line of poetry—an overture to the magnificence of the human body. I realized in that moment that women have no clue about our own beauty; no clue about the connection between pleasure and time;

no clue about this deep, delicious, endlessly replenishing source of divinity within each of us.

All these years I had been looking for the Goddess. Suddenly I had stumbled upon her—in the last place I would ever think to look.

She was here, inside of *me*.

I was overcome with the experience of radiance that had been inside of me all these years, but which I had never known how to access.

I was the promise of womanhood that had come for me all those years ago, as I lay in my little-girl bed, lashes scraping the pillowcase.

She wasn't in a church, a temple, the Holy Land. She was here, in me, released from bondage by my decision to create pleasure for myself. I was overwhelmed. And I knew instantly that here, right here, was my mission: to draw women's attention to Her within themselves; to help each woman locate *herself* as the source of power and love and acceptance that we all long for.

That golden buttery caramel feeling continued to inhabit me, and to grow, as I lay on my bed and stroked my body. I was delighted by how much pleasure I was able to experience by simply touching myself. I tried different strokes—from very light and delicate to very heavy and deep. I touched every part of me, exploring the pleasures of my throat, my neck, the delicate skin on the inside of my arm that yearned for a light, airy touch. How running my fingers over my lips caused an electrical current to run through my whole body, giving me delicious chills. I touched my pubic hair, my belly, my sweet, pink-nippled breasts, admiring the beauty and the responsiveness of my body. I was overwhelmed and so delighted with the feeling. I was a wonderland—and I had never known!

I was instantly committed to teaching women what I had just discovered. I knew that in this place lay the connection between the Goddess (spirit) and the Body (woman). Sensuality was the portal for the Divine Feminine. I was embodying the experience of the Goddess who had come to me when I was a little girl. I just knew, deep in that eternal place of knowing, that this was the way.

I had had no idea that the Goddess was *me*—she was in me, created by me, and had always been inside me. I thought I would find Her in one of the churches, the temples, the shrines I had visited. I thought she was somewhere *out there*. I never ever, ever suspected that she was right *here* all along.

Casting the Spell of Rapture

The experience of one's own divinity is not an intellectual occurrence. It is not something someone else can give you. It is a bodily experience that—for a woman—is activated when she is turned on. *Turn-on* happens when she takes pleasure from her body, which is an experience that women have been taught to avoid for the last 5,000 years. We've been held hostage by a patriarchal culture that devalues turn-on and uses women's erotic brilliance in service to the masculine. Yet the erotic is where a woman's confidence lives, where her power is sourced, where she connects to her deepest feelings and longings.

I now know that all it takes to experience the Goddess—the meeting point between the human and the divine—is to cast a spell of *rapture*.

WHAT IS TURN-ON?

It's inevitable—every year in our School of Womanly Arts Mastery program, some wonderful woman gets on the microphone with a furrowed brow and asks me what *turn-on* actually means. Does it mean you're down to fuck every second of every single day? Does it mean you have to wear low-cut tops and short skirts all the time?

What this means, first of all, is that this woman has not yet experienced the kind of turn-on I'm talking about. If you know this turn-on from the inside out, you know it's not tied to any external behaviors or circumstances. It's a state of being on the inside. It might inspire you to dress more sexy, because it puts you in more approval of your body. It might inspire you to flirt with people, because it feels so good that you want to pass it along. But to avoid any confusion at all, here is a short explanation of what turn-on does, and doesn't, mean.

Turn-on DOESN'T mean:

- You feel like having sex all the time

- Your pussy is drippy all the time

- You're obsessively thinking about your pussy, or sex, all the time

- You have to dress in anyone else's definition of "sexy"

Turn-on DOES mean:

- You feel a sense of your own aliveness and your life force

- You know that your spirit and your body are one

- Your native enthusiasm is intact

- Your ability to reach for pleasure is on—especially when it seems difficult

- You're in your right mind and your highest power

- You're you—full, complete, and whole

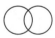

The sensation called rapture lives inside every woman. Rapture is the experience of divinity felt in the body. Your life force/spirit inhabits every cell of you. You are plugged into the Great Pussy in the Sky—what I like to call your GPS. It is the same as that feeling of divinity I felt when the Goddess came to me as a child. When you feel rapture, you get turned on—and become radiant as a result. I will use the words *rapture, turn-on,* and *radiance*

interchangeably throughout this book, because they all point to the same experience. It's the experience at the heart of everything I do. Every course we teach at the School of Womanly Arts is carefully designed to turn a woman on, and to teach her to make her turn-on sustainable, over time.

Rapture itself is hard to describe. To feel rapture, you must be turned on. So you will see, there is an overlap. Like all things feminine, it largely defies language. It is an experience, a feeling that comes from being taken inside the mystery of life itself. But perhaps I can give you an experience of it right now.

First, stand still.

Now read carefully as I shower you with words.

Let them hit you like raindrops. Let them transport you the way the slant of a sunbeam sometimes can. Here you are:

Joy.

Swooning from self-acceptance, self-love, self-celebration.

Freedom.

You are a line of perfect poetry.

There is beauty everywhere in you.

You are magic.

No right, no wrong, no shame.

You are so cute just now.

The unbearable, magnificent, fleeting gift of this moment.

Ecstasy for no reason.

The sparkling collision of death—of life—of rebirth.

Rapture is having all of these feelings. About *yourself.*

There is no *right* or *wrong* sunset; each is just a different experience of overwhelming, drop-to-your-knees beauty. Every single night. Rapture is unique to you; it is the feeling of the Goddess in *your* body.

But.

Do not fear if these paltry words fail to open the portal and take you there.

It is no surprise if you are not familiar with the feeling of rapture; we have no access to this sensation in our culture. As children we are all, myself included, taught to fear and disparage the experiences that bring us there. Experiences like self-pleasure, which is often presented as wrong and defiling, or experimenting and exploring sensually with other children, which is considered aberrant.

Rapture is the space where you know the perfection of your being—that it's a privilege to be a woman, to be alive, to be given the gift of feeling pleasure with your body. In order to feel it, you have to be willing to *turn on*. And most of us have been taught to run from the feeling of turn-on as if it were the devil. So many have had that connection broken—as I did—by abuse or violence. Others sacrifice their turn-on to self-doubt or aging or humiliation. Whatever the reason, most of us stopped looking for the light switch a long time ago.

A FLASH OF PUSSY

But it has not always been that way. There was a day, there was a time, there was a place when the light switch of a woman's turn-on was sought after. It was prioritized, highly prized, even revered. Across cultures, spanning centuries. Over thousands of years.

Let me weave you a tale of a pilgrimage—an initiation, a rite of passage—referred to as the Eleusinian Mysteries. It started with the goddess Demeter, who was bereft and heartbroken because her beloved daughter Persephone was missing and presumed dead. The magnificently beautiful Persephone had been abducted by Hades, who wanted her for his bride. Zeus sanctioned the union, a betrayal that hurt Demeter further. She was so deeply stricken at the loss of her daughter that she wandered the earth in a state of deep depression and bottomless grief. This was problematic for the earth, as Demeter was the goddess of fertility and harvest. In her grief she had withdrawn her light, and the earth was slowly dying.

Demeter did not care. She gave up being a goddess and became a mortal, wandering the road from Athens to Eleusis, looking for her abducted daughter. Demeter swore that the earth would remain barren until her daughter was returned to her. She took refuge in Eleusis, disguised as an old woman. The two young daughters of the city's rulers took her in, and she met their mother. Being surrounded by this happy domestic scene brought the pain of her loss to an even more intense level. She became so depressed she was almost catatonic, unable and unwilling to speak. Everyone tried to cheer up their guest, but with no success. Until a goddess called Baubo, disguised as a servant woman in the house, got Demeter to smile by telling her risqué jokes. Then Baubo lifted her skirts and flashed her pussy at Demeter. Demeter broke into laughter, and was enlightened. She returned light and life to the planet, became a goddess again.

Demeter swung into action and demanded Zeus deliver her daughter from Hades. (Persephone was only able to return for six months a year, bringing spring with her, but that is a whole other story.)

For 2,000 years, in celebration of this moment of enlightenment and the return of light and life to the earth, initiates would make the pilgrimage from Athens to Eleusis. There, this outrageous pussy-flashing scene was reenacted. There is very little known about this initiation, since the people who made the pilgrimage were sworn to secrecy. But it was said that when they returned from the initiation, they no longer had a fear of death. They knew their own immortality and divinity. Just as Demeter was restored to life by the flash of a pussy, so were the initiates.

The Eleusinian Mysteries make up only one of several ancient legends of how the flash of a pussy brought enlightenment to the earth, restoring life to the planet.

Yes, I know. I was shocked too.

For 30,000 years prior to the emergence of Christianity, our ancestors knew that pussy was a magical weapon. As Rufus Camphausen writes in *The Yoni: Sacred Symbol of Female Creative Power*, the symbol of pussy was protective and healing, able to avert evil and give power. Pussy was source.

For most women today, the natural set point is not this degree of pussy radiance. Our set point is stress, self-doubt, self-hatred.

It's comparing ourselves with others and coming up short. What's normal for a woman in our culture is to inhabit inadequacy, not divinity.

So the question is this: How do we access the fullness of rapture that is our birthright?

Enter . . . *pussy*.

TAKING BACK THE WORD

"Why do you have to use *that word*?"

I hear this from women all the time. Pretty much as soon as I pull out the P-word, someone gets up in arms.

So before we go any further, I have to present the case for the word *pussy* itself.

If you get a rather unfriendly feeling when that word appears, I am not at all surprised. You are very likely in the majority.

To those of us growing up in our patriarchal culture, pussies themselves are terrifying. They are desired and defiled in equal measure. They are powerful, messy, mysterious, and unknown. We are warned that pussies are what men want from us, as a receptacle for their cocks. Yet at the same time, we are taught that they are utterly disgusting. They bleed; they push out babies; they have orgasms in capricious and unpredictable ways. We are told they smell funny, and we are sold endless products to rid ourselves of their pesky fragrance. They are often considered ugly and in need of grooming in order to be presentable. We women shy away from them, and our men do not understand them.

Having a pussy, in this culture, is way worse than being called one.

So when someone—I don't know, perhaps *moi*?—casually drops the P-bomb, it results in a historical and experiential reverb that is much louder than the word itself.

There's no doubt that pussy is weighty. She has a ton of baggage. And yet, she is the only word for me.

My life's work is a reclamation of that which has been defiled. Starting with pussy.

There is no woman alive who has not had her pussy defiled or discriminated against, in some way. Belittlement. Gender discrimination. Rape. Molestation. Income inequality. The necessity for Title IX. When a certain kind of unaware, bigoted man says the word *pussy*—as in, "I gotta get me some pussy"—we know we are in trouble. We know we are at risk of being victimized by the unconscious masculine, which does not have our best interests at heart. We also know any offer he might make will probably turn into a physical and emotional mess.

And yet we know we may find ourselves saying yes to it anyway.

For, like so many women, we think we are *obliged* to say yes. Many women have spent their lives watching their moms, grand-moms, aunts, and friends choicelessly support a legacy of submission. Many women have been taught since childhood that they are an object, existing solely for the enjoyment of men. This kind of man is looking at women as receptacles, created for his use— not as full, equal human beings with thoughts and responses that might be different from his unconscious assumptions.

"Pussy" is rarely used in celebration or support of our womanhood. We may be called a "pussy" as an insult or a jibe. If we hesitate too long, feel fearful, or appear too slow, we get the P-word hurled in our direction. The insult might even come from one of our own: we women have, ourselves, internalized the dominant culture's viewpoint that "pussy" is a proper insult. And how about the rampant use of the word *fuck* to describe the worst possible outcome in any situation? "You are fucked." "He fucked her over." "I am so fucked." "Fuck you!" Such invectives are not referring to the person with the cock, my dears. Make no mistake: those insults are motherfucking pussy-centric.

So why choose a word that is so weighted, so heavy, and so rife with strife to describe the star of our show?

I mean, there are so many sweeter, gentler words. We could use the word *vagina*, for example—except that it's physiologically incomplete. The word *vagina* means "sheath"—i.e., the thing a sword goes into. It refers only to the muscular tube leading from the external genitals to the cervix of the uterus. So the word *vagina* leaves out all the exterior genitalia—the outer lips, inner lips, introitus, and clitoris. Calling a pussy a "vagina" is kind of like calling a penis a "scrotum." It's only part of the picture. As such, it's both wrong and misleading.

Which is a familiar experience for pussy. She's been called so many wrong and misleading things.

What's more—and at the risk of being incendiary—I've found that women who use the word *vagina* are often not on very good terms with the part they're describing. "Vagina" is like using the formal voice. Like calling a woman "madame." It's not user-friendly; it does not speak of intimacy.

So what should we call it?

Lots of people are using the word *yoni* these days. Personally, I am not a fan. *Yoni* is a Hindu word, whose root is Sanskrit. I am not Hindu, so it feels kind of affected to me.

How about *cunt*? It just feels too harsh, even though the etymology of the word is pretty impressive. The word *cuneiform*, which is the most ancient form of writing, derives from *kunta*—which translates to "female genitalia" in ancient Sumerian. *Kunta* also means "woman" in several Near Eastern and African languages, and its alternate spelling, *quna*, is the root of the word *queen*. *Kunta* is also the root of *kundalini*, which means "life force." Pretty powerful, huh?

The word *vulva* is kind of cool, because it actually refers precisely to the exterior genitalia. It is, in fact, the correct anatomical word when you're talking about the outer and inner lips, clitoris, and introitus.

But the word itself has no . . . *schwing*.

Vulva. It kind of sounds like *Volvo*. A safe but very unstylish car.

Whereas something wonderful happens when a woman says the word *pussy*.

Try it now. Whisper it to yourself, or say it out loud.

Really—not kidding here. We are all researching together. Give it a try.

Pussy.

Again, please.

Pussy.

There—see what I mean? When a woman actually *says* the word *pussy*, she smiles. Or laughs. Or catches a fit of giggles. She feels naughty, in the best way. Rebellious as a kid sneaking into the cookie jar. For some reason, speaking the word itself is a ticket to a secret conspiracy of some kind of delightful inner knowing; like a secret handshake, or membership in a clandestine sisterhood with the map to buried treasure. We women intuitively get that when we relate to the word that has so long been banished to the obscene and pornographic.

When *we* are speaking the word, the weighty reverb swings *toward us*, rather than against us.

The baggage turns into proud history.

And there is an immediate feeling of reclamation, which is the first step toward actual reclamation.

So, dear reader, *pussy* it is.

RAPTURE IS YOUR BIRTHRIGHT

"Life, Liberty and the pursuit of Happiness." The phrase describes examples of the "unalienable rights" that the Declaration of Independence says have been given to all human beings by their Creator, and which governments are created to protect. For a woman, the pursuit of happiness must include her experience of rapture. And the only way to truly connect with the female body's capacity to feel rapture is through her pussy. When a woman owns her pussy, she learns about her body, her innate sensual potential, and her creative capacity. This is not pornographic pussy I'm talking about. This is pussy, pure and simple. Undomesticated pussy. Humble. Glorious. Knowing her place in the world. No doubts.

Native indigenous pussy. Human pussy.

See, when a woman is in a state of rapture, she is standing in her power. She is able to feel the full range of her emotions and to stop teetering in that nasty neighborhood of diminishment and doubt. She can feel her wingspan, which is unusual for a woman in a patriarchal culture. Growing up in this male-dominated world, women use about 6 of the 88 keys on our piano. Sugar and spice and everything nice is what we get to be. But what happens to a woman's rage? Her passion? Her lust? Those ivories never get tickled. And through this rampant neglect, they get really out of tune.

Sometimes exterior circumstances can fire up a few extra keys, like when her heart bursts open at the sight of a sunset or at the birth of her child. Another few keys might get struck if she is transported by the fun of sports or dance or music moving through her.

But the only thing that offers a woman the *full range* of her pleasure is the experience of rapture in her own body.

Our bodies were *built* for pleasure. How do I know this? Because function follows form. Why else would we have an organ that packs 8,000 nerve endings dedicated to pleasure, with no other discernable function? I'm talking about the crown jewel of the pussy—our teacher, our leader, our girl guide, the one who brings us home and expands us to our full range: the clitoris. When engaged, this little bundle of flesh awakens our dead places, ameliorates our self-doubt, connects us to our divinity, and replaces our stress with simple joy. Men have no such organ. (They have about 4,000 nerve endings on what is essentially a multi-tool.) Just as the purpose of your eyes is to see, and the purpose of your ears to hear, the purpose of your clitoris is *to teach you that rapture is your birthright*. You don't have to rely on a sunset, a dance break, or a man. Your body is capable of experiencing ecstasy any time you wish.

Eight thousand nerve endings teach a woman freedom, self-reliance, and an experience of her purpose in life. Eight thousand nerve endings teach her that her joy is serious business, and that for the sake of fulfilling the gift of being a woman, she must not overlook her pleasure. Rather, she must be guided and informed by it as she makes her way in the world.

When she ignores her pleasure, a woman can mistake her purpose and believe that her function is to enslave herself to her job, or live only to serve her husband, her kids, her family. This misapprehension can turn into a life where she is utterly starved for pleasure. She can waste her life in a perpetual state of anger and resentment toward said job, husband, kids, and family—or anywhere else she's devoted herself in hopes of fulfillment. The omission of pussy has created a legacy: generations of women who live as victims, always blaming others for our unhappiness and not knowing how to generate joy, pleasure, and satisfaction of our own.

The entire purpose of the School of Womanly Arts is to allow a woman to completely reorganize her experience as a woman, so that her pleasure becomes a priority. When she includes pleasure, she is able to connect with her most deeply held desires. She is able to live a life that is based on her dreams rather than the agenda other people have for her. In the halls of the SWA, she is able to meet the Goddess within, to experience rapture, and to learn the Tools and Arts that will allow her to connect with her joy and pleasure on a daily basis.

When my cousin Hannah took my School of Womanly Arts Mastery course and continued to use the Tools and Arts in her life, she let her pussy lead. She's had a happier, more fulfilling life ever since. Even though it felt awkward and dangerous, Hannah picked up the phone and heard the call. The *awkward and dangerous* feeling comes from a piece of patriarchal inheritance that has both women and men associate the sensual with the pornographic. We have all been taught to suspect, vilify, and devalue the erotic. It has been a sign of female inferiority, weakness, and contempt. We have been taught that only if a woman can suppress her erotic nature is she truly strong and virtuous.

But when we ignore or suppress that erotic nature, we accept the oppression of the Patriarchal World Culture (a.k.a. the PWC). We reject the freedom, rapture, and radiance of the Divine Feminine, which I have come to think of as the Great Pussy in the Sky (a.k.a. the GPS). Such was the case for my cousin Grace. She heard the call of the Goddess, but the ring was so faint it was easy to overlook. Like when your cell phone is buried inside the pocket of your coat, under a huge pile, on the bed, down the hall, at a Christmas party. It's just way too much effort to dig, so you let it go to voice mail.

But what happens then? When we ignore our pussy reality— our pleasure, our erotic essence, our true nature, the gifts of the GPS—and prioritize the values of the PWC, we start to shrink. We're like the Wicked Witch of the West after her encounter with Dorothy's water bucket. Our life force gets smaller and smaller and smaller. Everything in our world is disadvantaged because *we* are not present. Our *truth* is not present because our *desires* are not present. And our desires are not present because the only way for a woman to connect with her desire is to connect with her pleasure. Pleasure is the jet fuel that makes desire a reality.

When a woman doesn't connect with her pussy, the lights go off inside of her—and inside of her family and her world. A woman can't do her job of being a woman without her sensual brilliance engaged. She is working with a 25-watt bulb instead of the 100 watts that are her birthright. The reason women lag far behind men at Harvard Business School and other top institutions is not lack of brains or abilities, but because we are living in a crisis of confidence. Just as I sought the Goddess outside of myself, we women are looking for our confidence in the wrong neighborhood. We think we're flawed and we need to fix ourselves somehow. What we don't recognize is that the only thing we're missing is the sensual intelligence that comes from a connection to our very source.

But can we really blame ourselves? We women learn to doubt ourselves by the time we're five or six. At that age, I had already decided that the Goddess was something outside of me; I had pushed her into the periphery. Interestingly, it was around the same time that I, like all other little girls in our culture, learned that my pussy was unspeakable. So where must we go when we are finally ready to bring the Goddess back into our lives, on center stage, where she belongs? To answer her call, no matter how faintly we can hear the ring? To master the Womanly Arts—which is also mastering one's own life? Why, of course, we must go back to pussy.

Homework: GPS Hunt

The Great Pussy in the Sky is my word for Girl Jesus, Gal Buddha, Ms. Yahweh, Lady Allah, etc. GPS for short. Your inner divine. Because the GPS actually is our internal navigational device. For this exercise, you're going to become a Great Pussy in the Sky researcher. A spy for the Goddess. Grab a journal and a pen, and sit down for a few minutes. Record your feelings and responses as you begin this journey.

Step 1: Imagine walking into your favorite house of worship. Do you notice any signs of the GPS? Is there an equal share of "she" and "he"? Do you feel a balance between the masculine and the feminine? Do you think it's important? Record what you notice in your journal.

How do your discoveries make you feel? Do you feel included? Excluded? Happy? Sad? Indifferent? Angry?

Step 2: Do you experience the GPS anywhere in your life? If so, where and when? Is she in nature? In other people? At your workplace? In the presence of a new baby? In the arms of your lover? Whatever you discover, it's all good. Just take notice.

Step 3: What were you taught about being a woman, from your mom, other family members, the culture at large? What did your religion teach you about womanhood? Was it exciting to think about becoming a woman? Discouraging? Neutral?

Step 4: What does "femininity" mean to you? Do you feel feminine? When and where do you feel most feminine in your life? Or do you feel more masculine?

Step 5: What does being a woman mean to you? On a scale of 1 to 10, how much do you enjoy being a woman? What do you not enjoy?

Extra Credit: Over the course of this book, your viewpoints and experiences with the material are likely to transform in unexpected ways. As a committed journal-keeper myself, I suggest you keep a journal of your journey with Pussy. Journaling is a really good practice, especially as you are on a growth trajectory. It helps you digest your feelings and keep in touch with yourself. At the very least, bookmark this page and come back to this exercise after you've finished reading the book. You may be surprised by how differently you'll answer these questions on the other side!

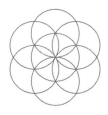

CHAPTER 2

RECLAIMING PUSSY

*Drawing and masturbation were the first
sacred experiences I remember. Both activities began
when I was about four years old. Exquisite sensations
produced in my body, and images that I made on paper
tangled with language, religion, everything that I
was taught. As a result, I thought that the
genital was where God lived.*

— CAROLEE SCHNEEMANN, ARTIST

    It was around eight o'clock in the morning on a very special Saturday. My friends and teachers, Drs. Vera and Steve Bodansky, had come to New York City at my request to teach a course called the DEMO. DEMO stood for Demonstration of an Extended Massive Orgasm, and that's exactly what was on the schedule. Steve was going to deliver an hour-long orgasm to Vera's body, right there in front of the class. Vera and Steve had just published a book called *Extended Massive Orgasm*, for which they were receiving a lot of press. I had organized their trip to New York and had enrolled the class and many private sessions while they were here. I had been studying sensuality for 10 years at that point, and teaching classes as Mama Gena for a few years (more on that later), and I wanted my students to be able to learn about female orgasm, just as I had in the early days of my studies. Students were flying in from all over the world to attend this seminar—and to have their books signed by the Bodanskys.

The Bodanskys' course consisted of a morning session downloading tons of information about the nature of orgasm, the study of pleasure, and the purpose of learning the very special extended massive orgasm technique. In the afternoon, there would be an actual demonstration of the technique, in which Steve would stimulate the upper left quadrant of Vera's clitoris with his index finger. This class was not a demonstration of sex. It was about educated stroking. Vera lay naked on a massage table, but Steve was fully dressed. His goal was to explain and demonstrate their very specific technique—a technique that resulted in an orgasm of a depth, intensity, and duration previously unimaginable. While the course was edgy, it was also exciting and filled with great information delivered in a highly accessible way.

Unfortunately, Vera had not been feeling well for several weeks prior to her visit. On the long trip across the country, she had only gotten sicker and sicker. We'd spent the days since her arrival going to homeopaths and chiropractors to try to get her some relief, but nothing was working. I finally called my friend Dr. Marco Santiago, an emergency-room physician, to come have a look at Vera. Within the hour, he had an ambulance at the door to ferry her to Beth Israel hospital. The look on Marco's face implied something serious was afoot. He told us he would be with her all day, as needed, at the hospital. As she was being taken out of my brownstone on a stretcher, Vera took my hand and pressed it to her cheek.

"You'll go on for me today, darling, won't you?" she asked.

Go on for her today?

Go on for her today?????

I knew exactly what she was asking. She wanted to know if I would take her place on the demo table. If I would get naked in front of a room of more than 100 strangers and experience a one-hour orgasm on their behalf. If I would step in, even though this group had specifically paid to see *Vera*, a well-known doctor of sensuality.

She was asking something of me that I had never, ever, *ever* imagined I would do. After all, this was *their* life's work, not mine.

When I started studying with the Bodanskys several years prior, I'd told them in no uncertain terms that I had no interest in training for a demo. I was interested in learning the techniques they taught for my own use, but I would never teach or demonstrate their work publicly.

After all, I was already Mama Gena—author, educator, and by now the mother of a four-year-old child. What if someone from my daughter's school was in the audience? What if one of my *students* was in the audience? What if this leaked to the press? None of my staff was certain if it was even legal to offer a course on this kind of material—much less deliver it myself.

When Vera asked if I would go on in her place, my mind screamed, "No possible way on earth!"

But somehow, my pussy answered instead.

"Of course I will."

Pussy had taken over the controls.

As it turns out, once unleashed and given a voice, pussy will take you places you might never have dreamed of going. In my case, she was about to take me somewhere *I had specifically decided not to go*. And with a speed and intensity that was making my head spin.

How did I find myself here, at this precipice?

How did I get myself into this pickle?

Why was this lovely woman even asking me this question?

What would my mother say, not to mention my *father*?

What I was going through that day might not be all that different from what you're going through right here, right now.

I mean, really—what are *you* doing, holding a book in your hand called *Pussy*?

I mean, I don't know you, but I'm fairly certain you're not *that kind of girl*. You've most likely been warned all your life *against* being that kind of girl. Or even *hanging out with* that kind of girl.

And yet here you are, hanging out with me—who's not really that kind of girl, either—taking a deep dive into pussy.

As odd as it may seem, what brought you to the point of reading this book is the same thing that got me to say yes to Vera that day. Something has called forth a part of you that *knows*. The power of the response within you might be surprising, even a bit overwhelming. But some part of you wants something here, even if that something is not possible to articulate. What you're starting to discern is that your pussy has a voice. That the voice of your pussy is distinct and separate from the voice of your PWC-educated ego, which is usually your dominant decision-maker. Pussy is where your intuition lives, where your deepest nonrational knowledge lives—sometimes known as your gut instinct or inner guidance. She integrates information from diverse sources, including the hypothalamus, neocortex, conscious, unconscious, and peripheral nervous system. This is why, when our pussy is engaged, we make better choices. We can feel the right next step in any situation. Women whose pussies are turned on make better decisions and move powerfully through the world. Pussy is truly our higher power, our no-holds-barred truth-detector, our way-shower, our leader, our divine director. She is, quite literally, our GPS.

And yet, we were never taught to listen to her. (In fact, we were taught to *never* listen to her.)

We were taught to run from her truth. (A.k.a. *our* truth.)

We were taught to ignore her and bow before some other god, some other viewpoint, any other voice but our own.

And we did as we were told.

PUSSY OVERRIDE

In this way, pussy became not the trusted inner advisor, but the force we were being advised *against*. The voice that needed to be tamped down, ignored, and annihilated.

How else would it be possible for 125 million mothers to stand by while their daughters undergo female genital mutilation? You heard me: according to UNICEF, more than *125 million* women have experienced the ritual disfigurement of their pussies in the world today. Allowing your child to be physically harmed goes against every instinct a mother possesses. Yet this practice continues to occur in 29 countries around the world.

Living inside a patriarchal culture, we women have had to make significant adaptations in order to survive. We have learned how to sidestep our deepest truth—our source, our knowledge—and follow the guidelines of the Patriarchal World Culture. For example, it would hardly occur to most women that they have the option to give birth at home. Yet for many thousands of years, women did just that—and quite successfully! Now it's way more common to hear a woman being persuaded by her physician to choose a scheduled C-section, or to use Pitocin to induce labor, than it is to hear of a woman who has a natural home birth with a midwife. About one in three births in this country is a C-section, which is a shockingly high statistic. Births are frequently scheduled for the convenience of the doctor, rather than the inner wisdom of the mother's body.

Meanwhile, our pussies are worth a fortune. But the fortune is most commonly made by the men who control them, rather than the women who own them. The sex-trafficking industry, which generates billions of dollars a year. Or an entire branch of Western medicine that exists to handle the "problems" of pussies. What about the vast fortunes we have forked over to corporations owned and operated by men, in exchange for feminine hygiene products to handle our bleeding and our fragrance? Or the drugs to manage our fertility and our monthly cramps? Or the senseless plastic surgery to reduce the size of a woman's labia? If only *we* could profit from our pussies to the degree that the PWC has!

We are taught to put the most basic aspects of our feminine power in the hands of the masculine. We are encouraged to suppress our strong emotions, our intuition, and our sensuality, and instead to be in service to the values of a culture that does not welcome our gifts.

The question is: how did we end up like this?

We each have our own story. Our story of how we were taught to silence ourselves—our voices, our instincts, our pussies.

My story is not so different from yours, perhaps.

I was born when my brother was 15 months old. My birth was a large-scale tragedy for Jonathan. It enraged him that he was suddenly forced to share my mother's attention. From the time I was three months old, he began to systematically attack me—and later, my younger brother, David, as well—punishing us for having destroyed his perfect happiness just by being born. We set him off on an unstoppable crusade of unrestrained anger and violence that ruled our home throughout my childhood.

When I was three years old, I began having fainting spells. As my mother tells it, she took me to Dr. Morris, the local pediatrician. She told him that I would pass out frequently and she was worried. He asked if I had any food sensitivities, or if there were any correlations between my activities and the fainting spells. She explained that whenever Jonathan beat me, I would faint. The doctor examined me and said everything appeared to be just fine, and suggested to my mom that her only recourse was to keep us apart and hope that I would grow out of it.

I did, but my brother did not.

He was an unchecked, unrestrained sociopath. He was older and stronger, and angry at everything. He spent his childhood committing acts of revenge and retaliation for my mere existence, and his rages dominated our household. The abuse was a part of what passed for normal in my house. No one interfered on my behalf, so I never fought back. I would just go limp and wait for it to be over.

Later in my life, as I was going through puberty, my brother drilled a hole through the bathroom wall, hid in his closet, and spied on me as I bathed. For months I felt something was awry, but I couldn't detect where and how the violation was occurring. I had a "feeling" that someone was looking at me, and I could hear suspicious noises. But it was only after it had been going on for months that the hole in the wall got big enough for me to actually see his eye. It was terrifying. I tried stuffing toothpaste in the hole, but he always bored back through to spy on me again. My parents did not intercede.

I was frightened all the time. I knew no other way to be.

My mother had tried taking Jonathan to the best child psychiatrist in Philadelphia when he was five years old, but the doctor evaluated him and said he was fine. My mother's response to his violence was to increase her own. I can remember her beating us all out of sheer frustration. She once broke a wooden breadboard beating Jonathan. My father just checked out and shut down, overwhelmed and ashamed. Here he was, a Freudian psychiatrist, with no control over his household. He did not seek help for us, only for himself, going to weekly sessions with his analyst for over 50 years. Meanwhile I grew up terrified and alone, in a sea of violence, completely cut off from the seat of my power. I didn't even know I *had* power, since—as sex-positive pioneer Claire Cavanah says, "Women learn to compromise before they learn to come."

Countless women and girls in this world experience violence and abuse in childhood—so many that this behavior does not even register as a problem. But every time a girl or woman is physically, verbally, or mentally abused, it furthers her disconnection from her power. She has no access to a sense of herself and no connection to her body, her divinity, or her radiance. She is no longer her own. She has lost her center, just as I lost mine. Her light has gone out. There is no one home, and no sense of where or what home even *is*.

My mother was unable to successfully intervene with the challenges in our household because her opinion was not considered as important as the opinion of my father, or the opinions of the doctors who were consulted. She had not grown up in a world where what she wanted mattered. She loved to sing and dance, and she was quite talented, but that was considered an inappropriate career for a young woman. So she became a secretary, a job she hated. She was once offered an audition for a famous band, but her family discouraged her from taking the opportunity. She decided to marry and have a family of her own, because that's what the PWC in the 1950s demanded. In the process she was pushing aside her deepest dreams and desires. To do so was a piece of cultural conditioning that no one had to teach her; it wrapped itself around every woman of her era like chloroform, anesthetizing her to her truth and teaching her to rely on the masculine for her sense of herself and her own rightness—which, of course, led only to more rage and disappointment. If the collective recipe for the American Dream actually bakes up a nightmare, as it did in our household, no one points fingers at the recipe. Rather it's the baker who ends up blaming herself.

But my mother need not have blamed herself. She, like all of us, was suffering from an overgrowth of the masculine, a common ailment caused by the PWC.

What all of us need is a dose of the opposite—a big dose of the feminine.

Masculine/Feminine Energetics

The absence of the feminine is the absence of *pleasure*. It's the absence of listening to our desires, our dreams, our feelings. In short, it's the absence of *pussy*. The feminine is the feeling part of us, our deepest intuition, our sense of community and connection. Additionally, it is a sense of spiritual morality and consciousness. The feminine is life. It may shock you to hear that she does not care about production, accomplishment, domination, assertiveness, or winning. Those are masculine values. On the contrary, she favors enjoyment, inclusion, surrender, and sustainability. The distinctions of masculine and feminine are not exclusively about men and women; they are primal energies possessed by all of us. It's just that all of us, men and women alike, have been indoctrinated to favor the masculine over the feminine for the past few thousand years. As a result, we are not very familiar or comfortable with her ways.

We need look no further than the headlines to see that violence flourishes unchecked when the feminine withdraws. I share my story of abuse with you not because it's unique. In fact, it's painfully common. Everywhere I turn, I hear of violence and abuse taking place in loving homes across the globe.

My friend's three-year-old son was sexually abused by his babysitter's boyfriend.

Another high school friend was forced to have sex with her English teacher.

My neighbor's two-year-old girl was molested at her fancy preschool.

Three of my four close girlfriends had experiences of nonconsensual sex while they were in college; all believed the rapes were their fault, and thus never reported them.

Two neighbors I had known while growing up were victims of incest.

And then there was me. I grew up in a squarely middle-class suburb of Philadelphia, Pennsylvania, in a maelstrom of violence, rage, and terror.

As you look around your life, you too will find stories of abuse—your own and those of others you know. Perhaps you never registered these breaches as abuse because they were so conventional.

Some of these cases will be reported, prosecuted, and handled with great grace and love. Perhaps there will be some redemption. But in other cases, like mine, the pain will be ignored, leaving a price tag a mile long for the bearer of the experience to pay.

My soul flew away from my body the moment I was abused. I was not me then. I split: out of my body, tucked safely in some ancient indigenous place, inhabited by all the souls of violated children, from forever until today. I no longer lived inside my body. I could watch me, but I did not inhabit me. I had checked out. I was homeless, lost, alone. And no one saw that I was gone.

Well, almost no one. For the Goddess saw me.

She's seen you too. In her invisible way, she collects those of us who have had to check out due to circumstances beyond our control.

This is a good thing.

Wherever you went, Sister, with whatever challenges you had to endure, I was there. You did not know me. I did not know you. But I was there by your side, and you by mine.

And we were hanging out, waiting.

For this moment.

To understand.

To receive the gift, the invitation, and the power.

The dazzling opportunity of being cast out of the Patriarchal World Culture and into the hands of the great transformer: Pussy.

DESTINATION: PLEASURE

Where will your pussy lead you, once you toss her the keys and allow her to drive?

Turning on your pussy takes you both forward and backward in time.

You connect to the raw joy and enthusiasm you had as a child. An unstoppably enthusiastic and joyful part of you plugs back in. Your sensuality and eroticism ignite, shining a sacred light on your deepest longings and desires. Too long pushed aside, they come front and center—forming the road map to a life that's a living, breathing work of art. A loving tribute to your higher power.

Awesome, right?

Yes, and it comes at a price: your membership in the PWC.

For your pussy will want to take you places and have you do things that are not PWC-approved. And since you've been living in that culture for so long, *you* will not approve either. Like when Vera asked me to perform the demo for her. The part of me I used to call "I"—who could never, ever imagine saying yes to such a request—was now replaced with an "I" who was unrecognizable to me. I didn't even *want* this new, fearless "I." Yet I was compelled by a deeper part of myself, one that yearned to emerge after so long in hiding. This part of me overrode my PWC-approved ego.

The ego is the part of us that whispers our fears. "I can't." "I am not good enough." "I shouldn't." It's the ego that makes us feel shame, self-doubt, and inadequacy. The only way to turn down the volume on our egos is to turn up the volume on our pussy. Pussy is the part of us that whispers our desires. She might whisper something like, "Get in there and ask for the raise you deserve," or "You are absolutely *not* too old to date that gorgeous young man who is interested in you," or "You have to quit that job you hate and write the book you want to write." Because pussy is the source of pleasure. And pleasure—especially orgasm—is kryptonite to the ego. The more pleasure you have, the more flush and strong your pussy voice becomes. And the stronger your pussy voice becomes, the more likely you are to connect with your power and confidence—and move in the direction of your most deeply held desires.

Why is pleasure at the center of everything? It's physiological. The unique design of the core of a woman's sensuality is the clitoris. And as we've seen, the interesting thing about a clit is that it has only one purpose: with its remarkable *8,000* nerve endings, it exists purely to produce pleasure in a woman's body.

Pleasure shifts your chemistry. In the presence of something pleasurable, the brain releases four "feel good" chemicals: endorphins, oxytocin, serotonin, and dopamine. These overpower the "feel bad" chemical, cortisol. When this happens, it shifts the balance of power inside of you. When a woman feels truly good inside, her confidence skyrockets and her sense of shame vaporizes, making way for her to live more powerfully than she could have imagined. Women have lived in fear, anger, and shame for so long, it's difficult to imagine another way. Pleasure slingshots a woman into a new paradigm.

Whenever we have a pleasurable experience, it increases blood flow and releases nitric oxide, which in turn boosts production of neurotransmitters like beta-endorphins. These beauties dull pain and create a feeling of euphoria—letting us deal more effectively with stress. When you have an orgasm, the main chemical players are dopamine, the reward hormone; prolactin, the hormone of satiation; and oxytocin, the cuddle hormone. Additionally, the stimulant phenylethylamine (PEA) is involved, which is also present in cocoa and chocolate. It elevates energy, mood, and attention. During orgasms, our brains are flooded with information, both from our psyches and from the nerves in our genital region. There are millions of nerve endings on the clitoris, labia, vaginal opening, penis, testes, and perineum, all of which feel highly pleasurable when stimulated and aroused. When stimulated successfully, these nerves send messages to the pleasure center of the brain, the same part of the brain that lights up when we eat something delicious like dark chocolate. Self-help and therapy are nice, but they don't accomplish a chemical shift. Pleasure is the direct antidote to the crisis of confidence and powerlessness women are currently experiencing. The journey from victim to heroine is only possible through it.

If, on the other hand, a woman neglects to create pleasure in her life, the body produces stress hormones such as cortisol, epinephrine, and norepinephrine. These hormones restrict blood flow, and nitric oxide levels plummet as a result. The consequence? Fewer neurotransmitters—which translates to increased depression, irritation, sadness, loneliness, and anger. There are also serious health risks: higher levels of cortisol in the body can suppress the immune system and decrease libido. Cortisol interferes with learning and memory. It lowers immune function and bone density, increases blood pressure, raises cholesterol, and causes weight gain and heart disease.

After studying sensuality for so many years, I'd taken myself from a sensual wasteland to the land of milk and honey. My frozen shyness had been replaced by confidence and joy. Instead of listening to my ego—the voice of the inner patriarchy that had shut me down for so many years—I could hear my raw pussy truth. And that led me to experiences that expanded my life in wonderful ways. Pussy allowed me to follow my own story line and live my unfolding dreams and desires.

Which is what we all want. We want experiences that continually break us and remake us into the radiant, powerful, erotic women we were born to be. We have been conditioned to believe that people outside of ourselves—teachers, parents, husbands, or priests and rabbis—will do that for us, more powerfully than we could do it on our own. But how could anyone do it better than we women can do it ourselves? We each have the divine inside of us, the Goddess within. She wants to have her voice, her choice, her day in the sun. Pussy has been buried under 5,000 years of patriarchal conditioning, but thankfully she is ready to reemerge.

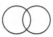

PUSSY CONSULT

One of my students had an interesting and valuable approach to turning up the volume on her pussy. After ignoring her for three decades, it was not easy to hear her pussy speak. So she purchased a puppet of a pussy and placed it on her bed. She would actually consult with it in the morning, before she went about her day. "Pussy, do you want to wear the red dress or the blue?" "Pussy, do you want to go out tonight or stay in?" Speaking out loud to a representation of an actual pussy helped her feel into her truth. Over time she learned her own perspectives and points of view. It became much easier to speak her opinions in the world once she had located them for herself. If you don't want to buy a pussy puppet, you can do the same kind of check-in with a hand mirror, consulting your own actual pussy. Or you can simply rest your hand right on her, while asking the question.

Need a pussy puppet of your own? See the Further Resources section at the back of the book.

This is why something so remarkable happens when a woman begins to *turn back on* and *tune back in*. When she connects to her pussy, she becomes an unstoppable force. Not through violence or domination, but through continually connecting to an ever-expanding sense of meaning and purpose. Meaning and purpose brought to her when she follows the true design of her life, charted by her most deeply held desires.

Kind of like the way you just trust a tree to grow. Once planted in her very own pussy, a woman begins to grow.

She learns she can deeply trust herself. She pays attention to her desires and treats them as her road map.

Indecision vaporizes.

She can truly feel her deep *yes* and her deep *no.*

She relaxes into the unknown rather than forcing or muscling her way through life.

She knows she can handle obstacles and understands that each one forces her to expand in new ways.

She connects with her deep indigenous beauty, no matter her age or outer appearance.

She experiences the divine in everything, especially herself.

She connects to her own internal GPS.

The very life force she was warned against becomes her most intimate guide and companion—the most count-on-able, trustworthy aspect of her life.

Sound too good to be true? Let's see for ourselves.

I want to invite you to join me in a little research project. Through the rest of this book, I invite you to become what I think of as a Pleasure Researcher. What do I mean? I mean *to take this book on as a research project.* As an experiment in your own experience. Try the exercises I'm offering, some of which might seem strange at first. (Let's be honest—they may not just *seem* strange, they may actually *be* strange.) But as a Pleasure Researcher, let yourself not be stopped or put off by trying something new. You are, after all, a researcher. A pussy scientist of sorts. Be willing to throw yourself into an exercise or an experience simply to see if the results are beneficial to you. Let your scientific curiosity take over; check your judgment at the door; and tabulate the results of your experiment. What do you have to lose?

So let's do an experiment. Our first bit of pleasure research.

I want you to ask her these questions, right now:

Pussy, darling, do you feel relieved that I am paying closer attention?
Do you feel happy that we are chatting?
Are you pleased I am offering you a chance to be heard?
Can you feel her answer?

Think about your pussy. Yes, put your thoughts right there, at the meeting of your thighs. (Even just thinking about her starts the feel-good chemicals flowing.) Now what do you feel?

It might be a light pulsing.

A throb, perhaps.

Or simply a sense of lightness.

A heightened awareness.

This is a gorgeous and excellent beginning. There will be more to come.

For the more you trust her, the more she will learn to trust you. And the more she will speak up at all the right moments. Like a good researcher, take notes. Journal your questions and her responses.

Homework: Pussy Rehab Sequence

When I first discovered the importance of pussy, I felt kind of ashamed. Even though I understood its value intellectually, I couldn't really feel her on a regular basis. I had been "dead down there" for so long, I was slow to wake up.

So I created a three-part Pussy Rehab Sequence to bring me back into contact. Consider this your first Pleasure Research project.

Step 1. Get in touch. On the first day of your Rehab, set the timer on your phone to go off once every hour. Each time you hear that chime, rest your hand on your pussy. Over or under your clothes, however is easiest for you. Keep your hand in place for at least 60 seconds. As you do, simply notice her. Notice what you feel. Any warmth, any tingles? Let her communicate with you; notice how just being in contact will soothe and ground you.

Step 2. Go panty-free! Going without undies is another way get in closer contact with your pussy. This little tip gave rise to a tradition in the SWA community called Panty-Free Friday. Mark this weekly holiday in your calendar. It's your little secret—no one has to know. (Remember, it's all in the spirit of research!) You will feel energized, enlivened, and a little bit naughty.

Step 3. Say hello on the regular. Slip a hand mirror in your purse and, a few times a day, take a peek at your pussy. Greet her with, "Hello, gorgeous!" and notice what you get in return. You'll see—she *loves* attention, and giving it will make *you* feel wonderful. Start each day with "Good morning, beautiful!" and watch your day unfold with grace and ease. Go to bed with a "Sleep well, sexy!" and you'll drift off sweetly into the land of nod.

Practice this Pussy Rehab Sequence for at least three weeks, and notice the differences you feel. How did your first research project go? Please write this up in your journal.

THE FIVE STAGES OF PUSSY

It was because I had turned on and tuned in to my own pussy voice that I croaked out a "yes" that day to Vera. It was because of pussy that I headed downtown to the SoHo loft where the demo was taking place.

Curiously, I was not nervous—just excited and energized, like a racehorse before a race. By this point in my sensual journey, I knew my body well. I knew my capacity to feel. I had fully taken on the project of awakening and exploring my 8,000 nerve endings. I knew how to experience orgasm with every cell of my being. I had trained my body—through literally thousands of hours of stroking sessions—to experience orgasmic sensation from the very first stroke I received. I had developed an unexpected confidence in my pussy and her capacity to experience pleasure.

So that day, even though I had never done a demo before, I knew I was ready. I knew that I knew how to *come*.

I *knew* how to come.

I could never have imagined what a profound spiritual impact this would have on me. My connection to ecstasy and divinity overrode my natural shyness and hermit-like tendencies, transforming me into the joyful, exuberant, sensual being I had always wanted to be.

When we are separated from her—as so many of us have been, for many thousands of years now—we are separated from our life force.

But you got through the first knothole. Your ancient, indigenous pussy wisdom broke through the patriarchal wall of our culture, whispered in your ear, and you listened. Lucky you.

She is the greatest untapped natural resource on this planet, standing for the creative unfolding of everyone and everything.

Every single one of us exists because of pussy.

It's time we listened to she who made us all possible. It's time to celebrate the part of ourselves that has never been celebrated before. Time to bow before a new shrine. Time to reconsecrate a long-desecrated altar. Time to reclaim the heart and soul of your life, the heart and soul of this book: pussy.

When a woman first takes on the project of pussy reclamation, there are some obstacles to overcome. Because we have been warned away from her for so long, we have a sense that it's not *seemly* to take up with the pussy. Rather, we believe we should continue our long-standing disassociation from her. We wouldn't want to risk our reputation, would we?

In my experience, a woman's reacquaintance with pussy breaks out into five very distinct stages:

- **Stage 1: Complete and total revulsion.** *Bleh. Bleck. Yuck. Gross.* She finds everything *pussy* to be revolting and disgusting, worse than sifting through the garbage or cleaning up after the dog.

- **Stage 2: She picks up the mantle of the scientific researcher.** She is able to find a sense of curiosity and perspective from behind her conceptual white coat. She is able to tolerate looking in pussy's direction without nausea.

- **Stage 3: Her natural curiosity engages.** She becomes an affectionate researcher, interested in learning about the scientific brilliance of the design called *pussy*, curious about the variations and similarities. She suspects that there is an aspect of woman that will never be known to her if she does not investigate and research the gift of her 8,000 nerve endings.

- **Stage 4: She becomes a pussy aficionado.** A pussy connoisseur, if you will. She begins to take great pride in the landscape, the architecture, the potential that comes with owning a clitoral pleasure center such as hers. She realizes that a woman who owns her pussy owns her life. Her relationship to herself changes dramatically; her confidence soars in ways she could not have imagined or anticipated.

- **Stage 5: Rapture.** Pure and simple. The way Gustave Courbet felt when he painted *L'Origine du monde*. (Don't know it? Look it up.) Or the way Mickalene Thomas felt when she painted *Origin of the Universe*. (Google this one for sure.) She sees, feels—*experiences*—awe. She connects to the power of being the portal to life itself. She wells with tears of gratitude and astonishment at the privilege of being a woman—the living, breathing gateway to creation. She hears Handel's "Hallelujah" chorus. She hears "Let heaven and nature sing." Or the singer Khia rocking "My Neck, My Back." (Check out the lyrics online—but not while you're at work!)

Suffice it to say, I want to get you to Stage 5.

I want to seduce you into trusting your pussy. Trusting and listening to your inner GPS.

It's what the rest of this book—and my life—is about.

My life took an even sharper turn toward pussy that day at the loft with Steve Bodansky. We explained to the crowd of more than 100 men and women that Vera was on her way to the hospital, and that I had agreed to step in for her. We explained that I had never done a public demo before, but that I had been studying orgasm for over a decade. We said anyone who wished could have their money back. No one asked.

I dropped my robe and laid back on the massage table, my legs spread in front of 100 people. For the next hour, Steve gave me an extended massive orgasm. It was amazing. I had never felt so much sensation, or so much pleasure. It was the opposite of what I was expecting: my pussy actually *liked* the attention of all the people in the audience. When you think about it, I was receiving everything that pussies love: attention, approval, appreciation, praise, and pleasure. I felt the unmistakable connection between me and every other living breathing person and everything on earth. I was the energetic current, the conduit, the source. I was the wind in the trees, the sunshine, the ocean waves. I was not only a part of the energetic fabric of the universe, I was a contributor. Me, who a few years earlier had been the most disconnected, disenfranchised, disembodied creature you'd ever met. Now here I was, sparkling like a sequined drum majorette leading the pussy marching band. I was not only the star of my own show, but from the pussy perspective, I could see that I had always been. Everything in my life had been leading to this moment. The Goddess in me was set free.

I was doing a favor for my friend Vera, but actually Vera had done the favor for me. She had brought me to a place so far past the shame and pain of my upbringing that there was no going back. I was free, and it was my pussy that had freed me. My gratitude was unending. I had been a woman divided from the word, divided from her body, divided from the world. But that day my pussy hurled me into a sense of radiant reconnection so powerful that she gave me enough juice to reconnect the world. Your pussy is longing to do the same for you. (Don't worry: following pussy won't necessarily land you spread-eagled in front of 100 strangers. That was *my* adventure. Your pussy will choose the perfect adventure for *you*.) That's why she made you buy this book. She wants you to connect with her—so that she can connect you to the world. She's nominating you for the starring role, rather than the best supporting actress. She wants you to feel your magnificence, to own your sensual brilliance, to inhabit the full landscape that she created for you. She wants you to experience the pleasure revolution in your own life. She wants you to know that we are all sisters, we are all creatrixes, and that pleasure is not only our birthright, it's our access point to the Divine. She is now, and has always been, the Great Transformer—and in the next chapter, I'll take you on a little tour of what she can do.

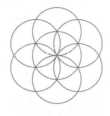

CHAPTER 3

THE GREAT TRANSFORMER

*Female sexual pleasure, rightly understood,
is not just about sexuality, or just about pleasure.
It serves, also, as a medium of female self-knowledge
and hopefulness; female creativity and courage; female
focus and initiative; female bliss and transcendence;
and as medium of a sensibility that feels very much
like freedom. To understand the vagina properly is to
realize that it is not only coextensive with the female
brain, but is also, essentially, part of the female soul.*

— NAOMI WOLF

So pussy is the source of our pleasure, and pleasure is the source of our power. Yet each year when I greet my new crop of SWA students I am facing a room of several hundred women who think everything about themselves is completely and utterly wrong. From the way they look, to the way they feel, to the bodies they were born into.

In the PWC, we women grow up believing we are wrong and broken. For me, it came after a childhood full of abuse—violence that was never talked about or intervened upon. I grew up believing there was something terribly shameful about me. By the time I was in my mid-20s, I had tried to solve the problem of my wrongness with therapy, self-help, and academic-style research—everything I could think of. But no matter what I did, I never got to "good." I never found the connection to my own joy. If you had asked me what the problem was, I wouldn't have thought to tell you about my brother's abuse. It was so much a part of my early life at home that it didn't even register as an issue. But the sense of being broken was what I woke up to every morning, and went to sleep with every night. I knew the last place I ever wanted to go was home, and the last people on earth I wanted to be with were my family.

I was both desperate to find that ancient connection to my native passion, and living with a deep, overwhelming hopelessness that it would never happen for me. Not in this lifetime, anyway, and maybe not ever.

I didn't realize I was in my "before." See, for every woman there's a "before" and an "after."

Before *pleasure*. After *pussy*.

My "before" started with my childhood of abuse and continued through my college years, as I tried my best to find a way to succeed in the PWC—all while dragging an overwhelming boatload of childhood baggage. In the years after college it devolved into despair, unable as I was to take any relevant steps in the direction of my dreams.

I didn't know why. I told myself I was busy.

And in truth, I *was* busy. Busy reading the work of Carl Jung, studying the archetypes, reading about ancient Japan, ancient Greece, Joseph Campbell, Merlin Stone, Marija Gimbutas. Teaching myself ancient Greek. Writing endlessly in journals, recording my every dream, feeling, thought. I had night terrors and I was afraid of the dark. I had no idea what I was so scared of, there in my tiny, quite safe studio apartment.

Looking back, I see that my coping mechanisms had finally imploded. My entire life up until that point had been an exercise in trying to look good, all the while hiding untold pain, rupture, and abuse. Not only could I not talk about what had gone on in our household, but I had to live with the extra burden of my parents' disappointment in me. I was not getting married to a Jewish boy, and I was not going to nursing school. They were not in support of the acting career I imagined for myself. I was not able to take the necessary steps to build that career because I was so ashamed of the paralyzing pain I was in. I could not handle their disapproval in addition to my own. Therapy seemed to make my problems worse: now I knew *why* I was broken, and who to blame, but it gave me no tools I could use to mend.

As a result, I crawled under a rock, hidden in the furthest corner of my cave.

And what saved me was . . . pussy.

THAT WHICH PLEASES THE GODS

Believe me, pussy was the last thing on earth I was looking for at the time. I had divorced myself from my pussy after breaking up with my college boyfriend. Though he loved me deeply, I just couldn't figure out how to enjoy sex with him. After a fun stretch of sensual exploration during our first year together, we started to have intercourse. I had grown up in the PWC, so I knew the deal. Sensual play was just for beginners; fucking was real-deal, advanced-level sex. This belief was confirmed by every sex book I read, every Hollywood movie I watched that featured a woman moaning in ecstasy during penetration. So when the time came for us to have intercourse, I imitated what I saw. I forced both of us to give up sensual play and skip straight to penetration every time.

In the process, I ruined our sex life.

I didn't enjoy pure penetration. But rather than following my pussy back to sensual play, I decided something was wrong with *me*. I broke up with this perfectly wonderful man because of my concept of *what sex was supposed to be*. At first I wondered if I batted for the other team. I experimented with having a girlfriend. Discovering that dating a woman was no less complicated, I decided to ignore sex altogether. I masturbated occasionally, but mostly I let my body go dark.

I didn't think there was a solution to my broken despair. And I certainly had no idea that the solution was as close as my own genitals. But then I went to that Basic Sensuality class and found myself dropped right in the middle of my own pleasure research. Simultaneously and "coincidentally," my historical research was turning up a precedent for pussy-as-savior. In my study of the ancients, I was discovering that pussy has long been the uncaped crusader. In mythologies across several different cultures, she had been saving the world from devastation for many thousands of years.

For example, I read about an old Shinto ritual that is still celebrated annually in Japan. During this sacred rite, a dancing priestess exposes her pussy in full view of the congregants. According to Rufus Camphausen in *The Yoni: Sacred Symbol of Female Creative Power*, this ritual is called the *kagura,* or "that which pleases the gods." It commemorates the story of Amaterasu and Ama-no-Uzume. Amaterasu is the Shinto sun goddess, the "heavenly shining one." She is the most important deity in Japan's pantheon of gods and goddesses. Every emperor and empress, including the current one, traces their lineage back to Amaterasu.

According to the ancient myth, this goddess of sunlight and life had been physically and sexually assaulted by her brother, Susanoo. Susanoo, the storm god—known as "the impetuous male"—had wrecked Amaterasu's heavenly fields, voided himself in her palace, and struck Amaterasu's vulva with a spindle shaft, piercing it. She was emotionally devastated, deeply betrayed, angered, depressed, and in physical pain. She was so deeply wounded that she left the world, wanting no part of it. She retired to her cave and refused to come out.

Reading this, my heart beat loudly in my chest. It was uncanny how close Amaterasu's experience was to my own. The years of abuse at the hands of my brother; the withdrawal into hiding. I could feel the goddess's pain in every cell of my being. Her hiding was *my* hiding. Her abuse, my abuse.

The consequence of Amaterasu's absence was that life on earth began to literally wither and die. The other gods and goddesses realized the grave danger the earth was in, absent her gifts. They gathered at the door of her cave and pleaded with her to return to humanity.

But Amaterasu refused their call. She was too broken, too devastated by her brother's assault. Not even the God of Wisdom could figure out how to solve the problem. One by one, each god and goddess tried his or her best to lure her out. But to no avail.

That is, until it was Ama-no-Uzume's turn.

Ama-no-Uzume, the "dread female of heaven," found the magic formula to lure Amaterasu out of hiding. How did she do it? Well, she gathered all the deities around her, not far from Amaterasu's cave. Then she began to dance the dance of life. In a moment of inspiration—like Baubo flashing Demeter in the Greek myth—she lifted her skirts and exposed her sacred pussy ("heavenly gate" in Japanese) for all the gods and goddesses to see. A huge roar of laughter and joy erupted, with everyone clapping their hands in celebration. From the depth of her cave, Amaterasu heard the ruckus. She could not understand how there could be celebration and laughter going on. All life was dying, and darkness had fallen over the earth! She crept out of her cave to see what had brought about such a turn of events.

When she did, what met her was a vision of Ama-no-Uzume's naked pussy. Immediately Amaterasu was caught up in the unleashed joy and ecstasy of the dance. With such a dance, how could she hide in her cave again? And so light and life were restored on earth, by nothing other than the flash of a pussy.

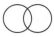

THE SACRED IN THE PROFANE

The story of Amaterasu and Ama-no-Uzume is reenacted every year in Japan's Kagura festival. This festival—and the underlying myth—have also given way to a modern ritual dance known as *tokudashi*. This unique dance is performed in the red-light districts of cities such as Kyoto, Osaka, and Tokyo. It is unlike any performance found elsewhere in the world. Neither conventional striptease nor burlesque nor peep show in the Western sense, it is more or less an ancient myth in a modern disguise. Picture a small brothel or dance club, and a stage full of women dressed in kimonos—naked underneath. According to Ian Buruma, author of *Behind the Mask*, "The girls shuffle over to the edge of the stage, crouch, and, leaning back as far as they can, slowly open their legs just a few inches from the flushed faces in the front row. The audience . . . leans forward to get a better view of this mesmerizing sight, this magical organ, revealed in all its mysterious glory. The women . . . slowly move around, crablike, from person to person, softly encouraging the spectators to take a closer look. To aid the men in their explorations, they hand out magnifying glasses and small hand-torches, which pass from hand to hand. All the attention is focused on that one spot of the female anatomy; instead of being the humiliated objects of masculine desire, these women seem in complete control, like matriarchal goddesses."

This outrageous, almost unimaginable practice is the only way an ancient sacred ritual can squeeze its way into contemporary culture. Why? Because we've relegated pussy to the profane and the pornographic. Today we do not know the connection between pussy and healing. In our world pussies are considered a receptacle, objectified for the use and service of men. This is the equivalent of using the Holy Grail to piss in. And the shocking part is that women have bought into this conspiracy! We consider our bodies to be shameful and wrong, and our sexuality to be shameful and wrong as well.

Let's unpack the word *profane*. Quite literally, *pro* is a Latin prefix meaning "before" or "outside." "Fane" comes from *fanum*, the Latin for "temple." So the word *profane* means "outside the temple"—which is where the feminine has been banished for the last 5,000 years.

At what expense? Only the life and light of the planet.

As a result of 5,000 years of patriarchal domination, there has never been more terrorism, war, destruction, corruption, and violence than we have today. And the countries in which women are the most disparaged have the most violence, abuse, and unrest. Indeed, even global warming is a consequence of the absence of the feminine, because all of us have been taught to *turn off* the characteristics of the feminine, including our innate capacity to *feel*. We can each ignore the "inconvenient truth" that Al Gore described in his film, because when we are cut off from our capacity to feel, we can more easily choose to turn a blind eye to the earth's need to be cared for and our own responsibility in the matter of caring for her.

Banish pussy, and light and life die—in your temple, your city, your country, your world. But just a ray of pussy light restores light and life to the planet Earth. Time to let her light shine again, wouldn't you say?

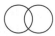

Plugging into the Source

Indeed, pussy had healed a goddess from the anguish of her brother's violence and abuse. I'm talking about Amaterasu, of course, but I'm also talking about me.

The pussy education I was getting in my More University classes was restoring me. It was healing me from the devastating hurt of my abuse—a hurt so deep no form of therapy had been able to touch it. Nothing else had worked. Not reading the collected works of Carl Jung; not studying ancient civilizations and languages. Only pussy could do it—and pussy did. Around this time, after many years of not dating, I met and married a good man named Bruce, who was taking the same classes that I was at More.

On the other side, I was not just *okay*. I was not just *fine*. No, it was as if pussy had launched me into an ecstatic experience of myself—an experience that had always been my birthright, and is the birthright of all women everywhere. I was remade, reborn; I'd been given back the life that had been stolen from me by devastation. I was suddenly reconnected with my natural, native enthusiasm—the joy I remembered as mine, from when I was a small girl. Thus restored, I wanted to tell everyone I knew. I began training to teach my own classes in sensuality, creating curriculum after curriculum, in hopes of bringing this incredible information to a wider public. Bruce did nothing but encourage me to find my way as a teacher. Eventually I started the School of Womanly Arts, a school dedicated to the work of the Great Transformer herself.

The School began with 12 students in my living room, but it expanded as I myself expanded. As quickly as I would uncover an archetype or feminine mystery and pop it into the curriculum, it would begin to rewrite me. My students and I would gain more and more power with every facet of the history of the Divine Feminine I collected. Every aspect of my life that wasn't "pussified" imploded and required complete re-creation. Right after I wrote my third book, *Mama Gena's Marriage Manual*, my marriage, by then 12 years long, blew up. Pussy had no tolerance for anything that was not in the highest good and integrity for all concerned, and I had outgrown that partnership. It was time for me to put on my big-girl panties and learn how to run my own life and my own company.

The unexpected benefit of this re-creation was that it required the School of Womanly Arts to grow rapidly. It was terrifying and thrilling all at once, because I had to grow rapidly too. I took the classes out of my brownstone living room and wrote the School of Womanly Arts Mastery program, which opened up the classes to hundreds of women, rather than dozens. This allowed me to reach more women than ever. But would this crazy leap actually work? I felt like Demeter must have felt after she was awakened by Baubo, and like Amaterasu must have felt after Ama-no-Uzume's pussy flash—turned on and inspired by the power of pussy and life. I wanted nothing more than to open the portal of Hades to the thousands of Persephones out there. Even though I was well-acquainted with the power of pussy in my own life, I had no idea what a ballroom full of that power could feel like. The force of pussy multiplied exponentially when the student body grew, and the results my students were experiencing were completely off the charts.

But of course historians had known about pussy power for centuries. Feminist historian Riane Eisler describes how our Neo-lithic and Paleolithic ancestors imagined a woman's body and pussy as a magical vessel. As she explains, our ancestors marveled at the way it bleeds in rhythm with the moon, miraculously creates life, and produces milk to feed its offspring. Not to mention the magical way a woman can cause a man's sexual organ to rise, and her capacity to give and receive sexual pleasure. Our ancestors believed that pussies were imbued with protective and healing energies. Flashing your pussy at the devil would frighten him and protect you from his grasp. Pussies could protect villages from opposing warriors, frightening deities, and wild animals. Ancient Egyptian women flashed their pussies at their fields, frightening away evil spirits and inspiring the crops to grow. Pussies were known to guard against evil and nourish both the individual and the community. There is a cave painting from about 8000 B.C.E. showing an energetic current emanating from a woman's pussy, extending to the hand of a hunter as he captures the daily kill. What this shows is that our ancient predecessors knew it was the Goddess—or, as I started to think of her, the Great Pussy in the Sky—who granted the power for a successful hunt. For it was understood that the taking of a life can only be granted by she who creates life.

In Catherine Blackledge's incredible book *The Story of V,* she quotes a Catalan saying: *La mar es posa bona si veu el cony d'una dona.* Translated, it means "The sea calms down if it sees a woman's pussy." Fishermen's wives would flash their pussies at the sea before their men would depart for a fishing trip, ensuring safe travels, plentiful catch, and safe return. If a woman wanted to invite a storm, she need only pee in the ocean waves. On the other hand, women from Madras, India, would soothe a wild storm by exposing their pussies to the storm clouds. In his book *Natural History*, the 1st-century historian Pliny the Elder describes how hailstorms, wind, hurricanes, and lightning would all calm down when faced with a naked woman. Plutarch, the ancient philosopher, describes how a large group of women, lifting their skirts, changed the outcome of a war. The Persian men were losing a battle against the Median troops and wanted to surrender. But a group of women blocked their way. Calling their men cowards, they exposed their pussies. Of course the Persians rallied and won the battle. Catherine Blackledge also describes how, up to the 20th century, peasant women in Western countries would expose their pussies to the growing crops of flax and say, "Please grow as high as my pussy." According to Russian tradition, if you are being pursued by a bear, a pussy flash will stop the assault. Our full-on pussy force field is more powerful than Luke Skywalker's lightsaber.

In my research I was thrilled and fascinated to see that the legend of pussy protection and transformation spanned multiple cultures, over multiple centuries. The discoveries continued. There have been more than 200 so-called Venus figurines excavated from a huge geographical expanse. These full-bodied female statues with gorgeously elaborate, swollen vulvas and lush breasts have been uncovered everywhere from Siberia to France to Italy, and date from a time period between 10,000 and 30,000 years ago. That's 20,000 years of pussy worship! It is interesting that only a small handful of sculptures of men have been found dating to this period. Cave carvings and paintings of vulvas have been discovered, dating from this same period. Clearly our ancestors worshipped pussy as the sacred portal to life itself.

All over Europe there are wonderful stone carvings on the sides of buildings—even churches—depicting the figure of a naked woman exposing her pussy. Said to ward off death and evil, these figures are called Sheela-na-gigs, and they adorn the exteriors of buildings in England, France, Scotland, and Wales. And all things being equal, who wouldn't want a little divine pussy protection? I sure did. So my SWA students and I began experimenting. We tried dabbing pussy juice behind the ears when going to a job interview, with incredible results. A few dots of PJ perfume before a date? It was like crack cocaine to a guy. When we wanted to feel powerful at an audition or a work presentation, we tried going panty-free. If we wanted to make ourselves positively bulletproof, we'd go panty-free *and* add some temporary tattoos, press-on jewels, and stickers to decorate our secret weapon: pussy. To our amazement we discovered that adorning her *activated* her. Like Wonder Woman's golden cuffs.

All my research of the previous decade was syncing up in my mind and body. I began to understand that women are much more than just the fairer sex, the weaker counterparts to men. We are not just here to reproduce on behalf of the male species. Women, I came to realize, are pure, raw, creative power.

Pussy became my higher power. My superpower.

I started unsnarling traffic by merely thinking about her. I asked for her help in finding the perfect parking spot and found one every single time—even in the heart of New York City. I would tap into my pussy whenever I was creating a new piece of curriculum and get an incredible download that both shocked and inspired me but played like a symphony in the classroom. Turns out pussy is not "a pussy"—she's a badass. I still remember the specific moment she said, "Divorce, now." Her timing was perfect, and I could not have made the move without her certainty. After my first almost unbearably rocky steps into the world as a divorcée, I have had the most creative and brilliant decade of growth—both for myself as a woman and for my company.

My pussy stood powerfully, like the dread female of heaven, when my daughter was seven years old and unable to read. Pussy first guided me toward hiring special tutors, then whipping her out of her "progressive" school and moving her to the best school in New York City for kids with dyslexia. What's more, she helped me get my daughter's expensive private education fully funded by the state. Pussy showed me the way.

One of my students, Fran, decided to see whether pussy could work at a distance. She was watching a football game with her husband on TV, and the Seattle Seahawks were losing badly to the Green Bay Packers. She knew her husband would be in a dark mood if the Seahawks lost, so she lifted her skirt and flashed pussy energy at the TV screen. Miraculously, the game turned around in the last quarter. It went to overtime and with one touchdown, the Seahawks won. After the game, the quarterback was telling reporters that "God is so good." Only Fran knew the truth: that God is impotent until the Goddess shows up to turn him on.

Yes, we are each that powerful. Try it yourself and see.

Your Pussy as Altar

It took me about five years of practice before I could say the word *goddess* with the same ease that I say the word *god*. Try it yourself, right now.

God.

Goddess.

Which feels more right?

Which feels easier?

Noticing is everything. We are willing to acknowledge that there are two sexes in the material world, so why not two sexes in the spiritual world?

It's all a matter of conditioning. Which is why there is such an epidemic of self-doubt and self-deprecation among women today. We have been conditioned to celebrate the masculine and devalue the feminine. In doing so we have lost touch with how to take exquisite care of ourselves. Why else would 23 million women worldwide choose to have cosmetic procedures every year—from breast augmentation to liposuction to Botox? Why would they submit to the knife or needle unless they believed that something about their bodies was wrong, bad, repugnant, or offensive?

Would we defile an altar, once we recognized it was sacred? I don't think so.

So how do we reconsecrate our own viewpoints in a misogynistic world? We must start with ourselves.

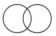

THE YONI PUJA

There is a secret Hindu ritual called the Yoni Puja, which is still performed today. In this ritual, the worshipper prays at the altar of pussy. A stone carving of a pussy is bathed in five ceremonial libations—milk, oil, water, honey, and yogurt. The object of this form of worship is for the supplicant to ask the Divine Feminine for whatever they need: health or healing for themselves or a loved one; financial help; fertility; etc. Upon completing the prayer, the supplicant ingests the liquid as a communion.

This ritual becomes even more interesting in some sects, where it is practiced not with a carved stone basin, but rather with the body of an actual woman—a yogini. The supplicant might stroke the thighs and belly of the yogini before anointing her with the libation, which mixes with her own juices before it's ingested. For certain rituals, a young yogini might be sufficient. But when the situation called for superpowers, the older and more experienced yoginis were much preferred. The divine sacred power of their pussies was more intense, as they'd had years to cultivate and strengthen their own knowledge and wisdom.

When I first read about the Yoni Puja I was shocked that such a practice existed. I slammed the book shut and could not open it again for a few months. It was too much for me to even conceptualize that there was a practice of honoring women to this degree. And yet how many times had a guy expected me to drop to my knees and honor his cock—unceremoniously—on a first date? How many times had I been with a man who felt no compunction to pay attention to my body but felt sure I would want to worship at *his* altar? He would not have had that point of view if all the women he had been with prior to me had not created or validated it. The patriarchy takes root inside all of our prejudices to such a degree that when we hear of a practice honoring that which has been so deeply devalued by our culture, we cannot help but recoil.

It's not wrong to worship the pussy, which is the seat of life itself. It just *feels* wrong because we are not used to it.

To see how bad our situation is, we need only look at birth in Western culture. After millions of years of trusting our bodies—and the help of other women—to deliver new life safely in our own homes, it's now considered normal to shut ourselves in hospitals. We place ourselves under the control of medical doctors who press for unnatural measures and schedule C-sections for one out of every three births. All of the power has been taken out of the woman's hands and placed firmly in the hands of her physician.

Which is more of a problem than we currently perceive. Why?

Because within the birth process is a legend. A legend of power and strength and resilience that every woman must learn. Whether it's the birth of a baby, or an idea, or a rebirth into a new part of herself, birth is the experience of a woman stepping into her power. It's not necessarily a pleasurable experience while it's happening. It's gritty and filled with effort and discomfort and doubt. But on the other side is a glory that can't be bought or faked. For a woman in the PWC, "comfort" means giving our power away to others. Discomfort is the experience of stepping into a new dimension of our power. Saying yes to the sacredness of being born a woman.

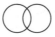

A woman's body is designed for creation. We create with our thoughts, our actions, our intentions. The body of a woman is the sacred vessel through which life gets created. It is a living, breathing altar. And what is an altar, exactly? *It is the meeting place between the earthly and the divine.* It is the place that is created here, on earth, to greet, welcome, and create space for the holy. It is a portal in this world, which opens into a world beyond. Each of us has way more than a drop of the GPS inside of us.

Through my reading and personal research I was beginning to see a woman's body as a living, breathing altar. We are the place where the human and the divine collaborate in creation. There is no human alive today who was not created and held inside the living altar of a woman. We have all heard that the body is a temple. But this is especially true for a woman. We need to treat a woman's body as an altar—to feed the holy in her—in order to live a truly sacred life.

What feeds the holy in a woman?

Pleasure, in all forms.

Serving her five senses with delight and beauty.

I found that when a woman begins to approach her own body as an altar, the results are transformative. When she gives her body delicious attention—like warm baths, with rose petals, by candlelight—she enlivens her own sense of holiness. When she makes delicious healthy foods, served with care and loveliness, she is feeding the sacred fire inside of her. When she dresses herself carefully and beautifully, she nurtures the best parts of herself. The more she bows before her own altar, the more glorious, powerful, and confident she feels, and the more generous she becomes with others.

Just as an altar in a sanctuary requires upkeep and maintenance to feel sacred, so does the body of a woman. Attending to her clothing, her hair, and her dress is not frivolous or indulgent or irresponsible. It is our sacred responsibility to look and feel as beautiful as possible so we can connect to the sacred within ourselves. To shine our radiance on the world. Why? If we disregard the sacred within us, we cannot connect to our ability to turn on. And when we are not turned on, we are not connected to our life force. And if we are not connected to our life force, it means we are not owning our own power. If we are not owning our power, it means someone else is. It means we have handed the controls to someone else—our partner, our boss, a parent, or society as a whole. The result is that we perpetuate our sense of ourselves as the victim, rather than the heroine, of our lives. We blame others rather than taking full responsibility. Victim is our cultural norm. It's how women in the patriarchy are raised to feel. We have not been raised to believe we are the source of our own power, the determiners of our own emotional state. But in truth, that's exactly who we are. All it takes to know this is to plug back into our radiance.

When we are turned on to our radiance, we grab back the controls of every facet of our story line. Powered by pleasure, our chemistry changes. It hoists us into a higher orbit, where it's easier to leave the victim and become the heroine. Turn-on is the ticket that launches us from loser to author of our destiny.

So you can see that self-care is a pathway to power. *Unimaginable* power. Power that is so sacred, so profound, that in certain parts of the world, connecting deeply and intimately with a woman's body meant enlightenment.

What would it take to get back there?

Pussification

For many years, I have been both teaching and living the experiment of connecting to my divinity as a daily practice. Some days I am better at it than others. Exquisite self-care is the easiest thing to toss aside when the mundane aspects of daily life take over. The world is designed to take the wind out of a woman's sails. To fill her with fear about all the ways she is inadequate. We each need the focus and determination of warrior women to fight the tide of self-hatred that comes from living in a culture that devalues us. It requires an enormous internal commitment: a commitment to treating the body as a sacred altar; to feeding our divinity a rigorous diet of pleasure.

To put our divinity at the center of our own lives is a sea change. Because in order to treat yourself like the Goddess, you have to interrupt the centuries-old habit of victimization. This habit is so deeply embedded that it's almost invisible, and certainly not conscious.

Take me. From the time I was very young, I was taught to not communicate my opinions. As a side effect, I learned how to be quietly resentful that I was not getting what I wanted. Did someone overtly instruct me in this behavior? No, of course not. I learned it by watching my mother. My mother, who was taught by *her* mother. Through this lineage of silence I learned that I was not worthy of respect. To speak up and ask for what I want indicates that I, and my opinions, have value. They deserve to be heard. To speak up means I must learn how to honor my opinions enough to voice them. To make this transformation, the practice of self-love was crucial for me. At first it was a practice—I almost had to force myself to notice, and then ask for, what I wanted and needed. But over time my perspective began to change. And so did my life. I transitioned from being small and victimized to becoming the force of nature I was born to be.

So how does a woman practice the art of relearning her own beauty? How does she begin to bow before what is and open the doors to what she might become? How does she reconsecrate her altar, daily?

The answer is simple. She *pussifies*.

Oh, yes, she does. *She pussifies every aspect of her life.*

Pussification means applying pussy values to yourself and your life. It means offering care and attention to make your world feel delicious. Your world is your temple and your body is the altar. In a house of worship, everything matters. It would not feel good to have a messy sanctuary or a run-down altar. Pussification is the practice of making every aspect of your life fit for the Goddess. Note that this practice does not necessarily require you to have access to royal coffers. You must be rich in only one thing: *positive attention*. Positive attention is what pussy values most. Yet we are so accustomed to giving ourselves *negative* attention: criticizing ourselves, shortchanging ourselves, doubting ourselves. Negative attention desecrates our altar. But we women have been giving ourselves negative attention so consistently, and for so long, that we do not even see it as a problem.

Too often we don't take the time to make ourselves feel good. We are so involved in making *others* feel good that we neglect to put attention on ourselves. Pussification is the practice of taking the time to do small (or large!) things for yourself, for no other reason than to make yourself feel good. It's making the space for yourself in everything you do. It might mean you clear everything out of your closet except for the clothes that make you feel hot. You throw out all the old, baggy underwear in your drawer, leaving only pretty panties that fit well. It might mean streamlining your kitchen, or clearing off your workspace, or sorting through your filing. Pussification sends a new message to the parts of you that learned you were not worth the time. It says *I am important enough to take time for.* Pussification is a practice, which means you do it whether you feel like doing it or not! You are a guerrilla pleasure warrior. Pleasure warriors pussify. Get it?

Each day I choose one small thing to pussify. Recently I pussified my purse. I made sure my makeup was in its own little bag; my keys were in their special pouch; my phone was neatly tucked in the inside pocket. Every time I reach in to pull out my credit card or to make a call, my pussy and I are happy. I have honored myself with my own magnificent attention. Not sure how to pussify? Think about what you, yourself, enjoy. What's good for the woman is good for the pussy, and vice versa. I try to pussify my medicine cabinet frequently, so the things I use daily are easier to reach. Everything is perfectly available, right where I need it. I put my Q-tips in a little silver shot glass, so they stand upright. My makeup bag goes right next to my makeup mirror. My little splurges—lime, basil, and mandarin bath soap and body lotion from Jo Malone—sit right next to one another. The result? Walking into my bathroom feels nurturing and loving, instead of depleting and effortful.

Some pussification practices have become daily rituals. I take a bath instead of a shower because it makes me feel more relaxed and beautiful. I use lavender-scented Epsom salts because they smell nicer than the plain ones. After the bath I use coconut oil on my skin; it smells beautiful and nourishes the skin deeply.

I have a daily practice of dancing naked (or in some hot getup) in my living room, to whatever song suits my mood. It helps me move morning emotions like crankiness through my body. If I am in a tragic mood, I might put on some Macy Gray. If I am in a happy mood, I might put on some Pharrell. If I am feeling unloved and unwanted, I reach for Lucinda Williams. Moving my emotions through my body is a way of honoring them, and honoring my design as a woman. We women are designed to *feel*, and to embody our feelings with love and depth. Rather than avoid the experience of feeling my feelings—which was what I was taught growing up—I now dance mine through.

Following my dance party, I sit at my altar for a small gratitude ritual. I have a series of stones and small objects I have collected over the years. I light a candle and pick up each of the 30 stones, one at a time. As I replace each one, I whisper gratitude to the Great Pussy in the Sky for different aspects of my life. I keep Post-it notes by the altar so I can write down any desires I have. Then I place each note in front of the altar. Finally, I might pull out my hand mirror and greet my pussy with "Hello, Gorgeous!" just to let her know I honor and remember her. Then I journal for a bit and write down not only my desires for the day, but the way I desire to feel. This helps to focus my spirit as well as my intentions.

My next move is walking the dog. As I do, I call a close friend and do Spring Cleaning—a spoken practice where I hand over anything that's making me crazy in my life at the moment. So within the first hour of waking I have moved my body, honored my emotions, connected with my gratitude, connected with my divine, dumped any negative charge I was carrying, and connected with my most deeply held desires.

I have, you see, reconsecrated my altar.

Homework: Spring Cleaning

You will want to do this exercise frequently to clean your mental closet of all the dust balls, lint, and collected crap from a lifetime of unfulfilled dreams and desires. When you don't clean out your closet—that is, rid yourself of all the clothes that no longer fit, the stuff bought on sale that never got worn, the old favorites that are too worn out to be seen in public—there is no room for new goodies. In fact, with an overstuffed closet you may lose your desire to shop because you don't have a vacant spot to put anything new. You might even have quite lovely things that you have forgotten about. Or things that were once lovely but are now ruined by neglect. This exercise clears your mind of all that old yucky stuff so it can be open and receptive to new desires. You might find yourself laughing or crying or raging during this exercise. All emotions are welcome. You can do this exercise alone—to a wall—with a partner, or with a small group of friends. I find it's most effective with a partner. Follow these directions and you'll have a clean slate on which to note all your newly recognized desires and appetites.

You both should first agree to keep what is said in the exercise confidential so that you can be free in revealing your desires. You are promising never to talk about the contents of the exercise with one another. Then sit facing each other, either at a café or some private place. One Sister Goddess (SG) asks the other the same question, over and over for 15 minutes. The other SG answers. Then they switch.

For example:

SG 1: What do you have on desire?

SG 2: I feel that I want my boyfriend more than he wants me.

SG 1: Thank you.

SG 1: What do you have on desire?

SG 2: When we were together last night he refused to have sex with me.

SG 1: Thank you.

SG 1: What do you have on desire?

SG 2: I love my new pink shoes I bought today.

SG 1: Thank you.

These daily practices are some of the ways I stay centered, grateful, and filled up with love and attention. Thusly pussified, I can open myself to whatever the day brings with the thick padding of self-love in place. This makes me far less vulnerable to losing my sanity when dealing with raising a teenager, handling a complex and lively office, being single and dating, and any of the other unforeseeable vicissitudes of life.

And I go further still. I wear clothes I love every day, even when I'm just staying home. I have figured out a simple way of handling my hair so it always looks pretty great. I have a brief makeup routine—a dot of concealer, lash curler, mascara, and lip gloss. It's easy to put on and makes me feel like I have some extra sparkle. Each of these steps requires a certain amount of effort, but the results are so worth the investment.

I am also conscious about what, and how, I eat. I try to eat as cleanly and healthily as possible (except for cheat day) in order to take the best possible care of my body. Perhaps even more important is the *way* I eat. I prepare my breakfast (usually kale and eggs) and sit down at my dining room table with real china and real silverware. I do my best to eat slowly and with gratitude. Taking food—which is a gift from Mother Earth herself—into our bodies and using it to nourish us is a sacred act. It takes enormous effort on my part not to rush, and not to distract myself with electronics, especially when I am dining alone, which happens a lot in my current lifestyle. Treating yourself like the Goddess is not easy. It is pure effort, like pedaling a bicycle uphill. But so worth it for the incredible view when you get to the top.

Every woman can, and will, design her own version of what pussification means to her. Your version of tending your altar might be completely different from mine, but the objective is the same. It's to create a wide landing strip for your own divinity so it can inhabit your day, your life, your body.

Homework: Pussification

In what ways can you pussify your life, today? How can you reclaim your beauty and celebrate the woman you are and the woman you were born to become?

To give you some ideas, some pussification rituals my students love include:

- Cleaning your home

- Canceling plans in favor of self-care

- Unscheduled time with a beloved

- Doing craft projects

- Movement classes (dance, yoga, etc.)

- Leaving plenty of transition time between activities

- Eating healthy, delicious foods

- Getting enough sleep

- Wearing sexy lingerie under your work clothes

- Drinking a lot of lemon water

- Adorning yourself with clothes you feel hot in

- Getting (or giving!) manicures and pedicures

- Spending time in pajamas

- Meditating daily

- Walking slowly down the sidewalk, as if it were a runway

- Self-pleasure (masturbation)

- Writing down gratitudes

- Reading positive books and articles

- Filling your home with smells and textures you love

- Wearing glitter

- Taking baths

- Setting daily intentions before leaving home in the morning

- Whatever makes you feel good

Use these ideas to inspire your pussification, or feel free to create rituals of your own. Journal how taking these steps to reclaim your radiance makes you feel.

The more we prepare ourselves for connection to our innate power, the more tuned in we will be. Tuning in is turning on. It's switching on our natural Goddess-given radiance. When a woman feels beautiful, and beautifully cared for, her radiance cannot help but shine through. Why? Because when pussy is happy, *we* are happy. Her radiant, transformational power—known and embraced over the centuries but forgotten today—is once again acknowledged, welcomed, and honored. Pussification is not a matter of vanity or self-indulgence. *Taking exquisite care of ourselves is serving the divine.* It is tending to the magnificent face of God/Goddess that every human being is. We celebrate our divinity when we honor our value and beauty—the value and beauty of our very own pussy.

Which is where we will go next. A guided tour to the center of it all. An up close and personal exploration of the star of our show. We'll take a look at (and perhaps even cop a feel of) our very own pussy, with a lesson in a subject we all need to learn but few of us have yet been taught. A lesson in what I call *cliteracy*.

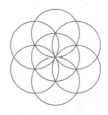

Chapter 4

CLITERACY

The Pussy Pledge:
I pledge allegiance to my pussy
and to the Pleasure Revolution for which she stands,
8,000 nerve endings, designed by the Goddess,
one community, under the hood,
with pleasure and cliteracy for all.

— Mama Gena

When you're lost and you know it, you understand that you have to find your way back home. You take relevant steps to do just that. You ask people who know. You consult maps. You turn on your GPS and get a guided tour right back home.

But what if you didn't even know you had a GPS? What if it was right there at your fingertips but you had absolutely no clue?

Worse, what if you had been lost for so long that you didn't even know you were lost? Because that is just the way things always are, always were, and—you figure—always will be?

That's pretty much the state of womankind right now.

We are so accustomed to hating our female body, so accultur-ated to despising the beating heart and soul of our femininity—the pussy—that we don't even hold that there might be another way to feel. *Women have no idea that hating ourselves is actually a consequence of hating our pussies.* We think we hate ourselves because there is something wrong with us. It would never occur to us that it might have to do with the way we feel about, relate to, and disown the core of our feminine nature. No woman in her right mind would draw a link between how we feel about our pussies and the fact that of 197 heads of state in the world today, only 22 are women. If we inquired as to why women run only 21 of the top 500 companies in the United States by revenue, pussy would not even enter the conversation. We wouldn't draw a connection between the fact that women have been taught that our pussies are disgusting and problematic and the fact that we hold just 18 percent of U.S. congressional offices.

But pussy has everything to do with it.

Thoughts become things.

Bigotry is a series of thoughts that become a reality.

For example, it often seems that many Palestinians don't even question that they hate Israelis, and vice versa. It just seems as if it has always been that way. To change your opinion would jeopardize your standing in your community. Your loved ones would strongly object to you having a different opinion than they do about their rival faction.

It's no different for women.

If I learn self-hatred and self-doubt from my mother, then I must adopt her point of view if I want to show my love to her. Otherwise I will be disrespecting her. I must hate myself because I love her and I want her to love me.

Then I continue the legacy and infect my daughter and my daughter's daughter with a viewpoint that I learned from my own lineage. A viewpoint I have never questioned, because it is baked into every woman I have ever encountered. Women spread the virulent condition of self-doubt and self-hatred without even knowing we're contaminated. It's kind of like a cold in January—everyone just seems to have one.

So how do you recover yourself from a long period of cultural amnesia?

How do you—as the poet Galway Kinnell says—"reteach a thing its loveliness"? How do you hold up the mirror to a woman's innate and eternal beauty when she can barely even meet her own reflection?

You do it through *cliteracy.*

Cliteracy is my fun and frivolous term for an incredibly profound and important process. It's introducing a woman to a deep body of knowledge about her raw, awe-inspiring pussy truth—and teaching her how to love that truth into reality. Teaching her how to be engaged with her pussy, every single day of her life. Cliteracy means learning the depth and breadth of the gift of being born a woman. It's learning what pussy has to teach us, physically and otherwise, so that we can live her truth in our lives. So that we can take our partner there, and teach him or her how to play our full 88 keys. So that we can truly become literate in the language of the feminine, the language of the Goddess, the language of the divine.

I first encountered the term *cliterate* about 15 years ago, from a student of mine named Vanessa. She'd gone on a few dates with a guy who, shockingly, seemed to know exactly how to treat her and her pussy. She was not used to this experience, having encountered primarily men who had no clue what to do to please her. Delighted, she proclaimed this new love interest "cliterate." What I noticed was that the more cliterate Vanessa herself had become—the more she lived into her own pleasure and discovered what made her pussy happy—the more she'd started attracting men who were capable of treating her that way. The outer world had responded to her inner shift.

As it turns out, cliteracy has to start with the one who owns the pussy.

Function follows form. The optimum conditions for a pussy to flourish are precisely the same conditions that allow a *woman* to flourish.

This makes sense once you understand that pussy is our higher power. She is our deepest intuition, our connection to our nonverbal, nonlogical truth. She is the place where our humanity and our divinity connect.

She talks to us. She will whisper, "I know you are running late, but don't take a cab—take the subway." We don't listen to her, and there we are, stuck in traffic, missing our meeting.

She's there when we get offered that amazing job, the one that will look so good on our résumé. But as we are leaving the fluorescent-lit cube-farm corporate office that made us the offer, she whispers, "Please, no. Don't do it. I hate it here." And we tell her to shut up, because this is the best offer we're likely to get. We take the job, and within three months we're on antidepressants and wondering why we can't shake the misery when our life looks so damn good on paper.

She's with us on that date. The guy's résumé is fantastic, but she sees something else. "Something isn't right. We gotta get out of here." We don't listen. Six months and three new cell phone numbers later, we're finally rid of the stalker.

Even in the realm of sex, we have not listened to her.

Have you ever been in bed with someone and started to experience pain, but not stopped the sex, even though it hurt? She tried to get you out of there, but you were not used to listening to her. You were more accustomed to listening to *him*.

Have you ever stopped your partner from pleasuring you because you had the thought, *This is taking way too long*? She takes as long as she takes for a good reason. She wants you to have the most pleasure you can have. She is not in a rush. She knows she is the most interesting, fascinating, and wonderful thing there is. She knows there's no better way for you and your partner to spend your time than pleasing her.

Have you been on a date with someone you're not that interested in, but fucked him (or her) anyway, because it seemed easier than telling the truth? She wants you to learn to speak your truth. She thinks it's the most important thing on earth and that's why she won't leave you alone and keeps tugging gently on your sleeve when you try to brush her away.

Has your partner ever tried to impress you with his staying power—fucking you until your pussy feels like sandpaper—and you've still moaned, "Yes . . . yes . . . yes"? Once again she refuses to let you think it's okay to sell yourself out like that. She thinks she is worth protecting.

We don't listen to her, but we should. Pussy *knows*.

As writer Natalie Angier says, your clitoris is a proper little brain. In her book *Woman: An Intimate Geography*, Angier explains how the clit gathers information from your conscious, unconscious, hypothalamus, neocortex, and peripheral nervous system. This "mini brain" tracks it all on your behalf, without you even knowing it. She has the ability to sense, discern, and intuit. Your ego might be fooled, but not your pussy. She can feel the truth behind the truth.

Pussy is your own built-in psychic, your own inner guide, your divining rod. You don't need to call 1-800-PSYCHIC, hire an angel whisperer, or put another astrologer on your payroll. Your pussy is all of that and more. Pussy can assist you in discerning your next wise steps, your next outrageous adventure, your next love or passion. When you are piped into your higher power—your very own Great Pussy in the Sky, living inside of you—you can move with confidence in the world. She knows you so well. She spends all of her time with her attention on *you*. When you're listening to her, you don't park your car in that deserted parking lot late at night, because it scares her. You might give that kind of awkward guy a second date, because something about him pleases her. You will turn down the aforementioned fluorescent-lit cube-farm job offer and take a lower-paying job at Starbucks instead so you have time to write your first novel, which eventually will make you more money than you could have dreamed. You will tell your lover what you like, and you will tell your lover what *doesn't* feel good. You will no longer rely on your husband's or lover's psychic powers to make you happy in bed; you will take the reins and steer, because you have done the research to learn how the reins work and where they want you to go. You will be able to show your partner what makes your pussy happy, what makes her sing, and what makes her moan.

In short, you will take control of your sensual destiny.

How? By learning your body. You have investigated what turns her on and what turns her off. You can sense what she wants, and you are not afraid to experiment. You trust her so much that when she says you've had enough, you have your lover stop, midstroke, if his cock is irritating or chafing you. You trust her. Just like you trust your appetite, you stop when you are full and you don't force yourself to have more than you want. (Except maybe a little chocolate now and then.)

You have become, in a word, *cliterate*.

Homework: Ask Your Pussy

Your pussy is your intuitive knowing, your higher power, your wisdom within. Use this exercise to let her guide you.

Step 1: Think of a decision you're making right now. It might be a big one, like changing careers, or a small one, like where to eat dinner.

Step 2: Now cup one hand around your pussy. It can be over or under your clothes, however you choose.

Feel her. Notice any sensations, and take note of them.

Step 3: Once you've made contact, whisper your question in her direction. You may say it out loud, or quietly in your own mind.

Example: *Pussy, should I go on a date with this guy from OkCupid?*

Step 4: Now listen for her response. Is it a yes? A no? Whatever you hear, you can trust it.

Just for kicks, do what she says. Record the results.

Step 5: Tomorrow, ask her for her opinion on another topic. But that time, do the opposite of what she tells you. Record your results.

Which brought you a better outcome?

Remember, this is all pleasure research. There are no rights and wrongs, no good and bad. We are simply on a mission of discovery.

Why We Need Cliteracy

Cliteracy is the core and beating heart of who and what a woman is in this world today. It is packed with all of her unpacked potential, pleasure, and power. Right now, in this world, we are up to our eyeballs in cock. And even if a woman is unfamiliar with a certain cock, or new to the cock game, many men feel pretty darn comfortable asking for what they want and telling her exactly how they want it. Women have never been encouraged to look or feel or touch or experiment or learn anything about ourselves. We have been encouraged to simulate Snow White or Sleeping Beauty—i.e., just kind of lie there and hope our prince knows what he's doing. We make sure our kids have driver's ed before we let them sit behind the wheel of a car, but we don't hear too much about moms teaching their daughters how to self-pleasure. Nor do we hear about dads teaching their sons how to handle a pussy. If we *did* hear of such a thing, it would likely register as horrifying.

We women have all been sworn to some kind of code of shame. We learn how to come by watching men get off, and then we judge ourselves as wrong because pussies don't work as fast, or seemingly efficiently, as cocks. We use the masculine as the standard, and consequently view ourselves and what we might want as terribly wrong and unimportant.

If we were to follow the rules of cliteracy, life would be very different.

There would be no abuse or violence in the world because we would all be encouraged to feel our feelings deeply and pay attention to the responses of others.

When we are tuned in to other people we cannot harm them. Cliteracy teaches us to tune in to one another, not tune out.

The porn industry would have very different content; it would be styled to reflect what gives a woman pleasure, as much as it reflects what pleases a man.

Hollywood would no longer have a majority of penetration-centric sex scenes. Sometimes it would be about her pleasure. Women would speak up, and men would listen.

Women would walk away from situations when they were being disadvantaged, hurt, or ignored.

Mother Earth would be honored, rather than abused.

The list goes on . . . and on.

A woman's body creates life, and yet we argue with it. We hate the blood, the smell, the gushiness, the wild hair, the vivid colors, the way it turns on, the way it turns off, and the essential brilliance of the way it operates. We are ashamed of our sacred creative essence, the seat of our divine feminine power.

Cliteracy is about educating women and men to the unimaginable majesty of pussy.

Just like with my student Vanessa, we cannot teach the larger culture to cherish us until we cherish ourselves.

Cliteracy is not only crucial in the bedroom. Understanding our own pleasure system is critical for the health of the total woman. Why? Because we are every bit as sensitive as our 8,000 nerve endings. What works for the clit works for the whole woman. Think of the clit as the instruction manual for woman. If you abuse the clit, she shuts down. If you appreciate her, she opens up. Same goes for a woman. If you want to learn how a woman operates, just learn how a pussy operates. It is one and the same. Women recoil when hurt or humiliated, and flower when we are honored and attended to. Men know it's important to protect themselves from getting kicked in the nuts, because it hurts. But women do not know how to protect ourselves from hurt. We have never been taught what causes pain or pleasure to a pussy. Our culture simply does not value it. Women will frequently submit to hurt and pain because we don't know that pleasure is our birthright. In fact, I believe that making sure every child is cliterate is just as important as making sure every child can read.

Cliteracy teaches a girl how to tune in. How to treasure—how to cherish—herself in a culture where she's more likely to learn self-hatred than self-love. Self-love is self-protection. Self-hatred exposes girls and women to all kinds of disrespect, both on the inside and on the outside. Cliteracy teaches boys and men how to honor and pay attention to women.

So welcome to the classroom of the clit. Sit down, relax, and enjoy your first lesson in cliteracy.

THE RULES OF CLITERACY

Cliteracy starts with taking our own temperature. But what we're measuring isn't temperature in the sense of hot and cold. What we're testing is our level of *turn-on*. Turn-on is our meter reader. Our litmus paper. Our truth detector. The pussy turns on when the rules of the feminine are being observed and honored. She turns off when we are being devalued or dishonored, by others or ourselves.

When I teach a School of Womanly Arts Mastery class, I start by asking what turns pussy off. My students are fantastic at answering this question. They know she hates to be rushed. That she shrivels when she is criticized, yelled at, or mocked. She turns off completely if we deprecate her. She hates to be threatened. She hates being ignored. She shuts down at the first sign of disapproval.

"And," I ask, "how about what turns her *on?*" The answers come less easily.

We women know what turns pussy off, but not what pleases her. Why might that be? The answer is simple: We don't know because *we have not studied what turns pussies on.* Cocks? We know all about them. We've studied pressure, speed, stroke. We've read books on the subject. But when relating to our very own center of pleasure? We've devoted precious few resources.

So the first subject I teach at the School of Womanly Arts is *pleasure*. We do research. We do homework. We investigate what makes her open up and come into full Technicolor. What we've discovered is revolutionary. Over my many years of teaching, I've found that there are a few key ingredients required when turning a pussy on. Literacy in these simple secrets is required of anyone who wants to please a woman. Pussy may appear complex, but her tastes are simple. Follow these guidelines, and you will be rewarded handsomely—in pleasure.

Cliteracy Rule #1: Pussy loves acknowledgment, praise, worship, and appreciation.

Pussy loves praise. Best if offered directly. She is delighted if your lover spreads your legs and whispers sweet nothings: "Your pussy is so hot. She is so beautiful. I love the color of your lips." A worshipping gaze turns her on so much. She loves her divinity to be noticed and revered. It enables her to connect with her own source energy and to connect her partner with his.

To increase her pleasure, all your lover needs to do is notice and report on her changing coloration—the deepening of her pinks, reds, purples. To mention the delicate sheen of lubrication that magically appears on her folds the more turned on she gets. To take note of the natural swelling of the clit as you get more and more turned on. Such simple attention delights and inspires her.

Pussies do not even need to be touched to be turned on. If your lover sends an e-mail noting how turned on he or she is just thinking about your pussy, you won't have to finish reading the e-mail before your pussy will be wet. Even if he is in Pittsburgh and you are in Nepal. Pussies love pleasure so very much that even the *thought* of pleasure is pleasurable.

Cliteracy Rule #2: She hates criticism, being rushed, being yelled at, being ignored.

Pussies are so sensitive. They can feel displeasure from across a crowded room. And if they feel your displeasure—or that of your lover—they shut down immediately. This is extremely important because there is no hiding with pussy. Not for you, not for your lover. If you are secretly worried that you are taking too much time and your pussy should just get off already, she will simply stop feeling. If *he* has the nerve to rush you or hurry her along, or appears in any way impatient or bored, then she will turn off the lights and close up shop.

If he is only interested in his pleasure and pays no attention to hers, she will get pissed off and lose any interest in turning on or opening up to him. The reason there is so much so-called sexual dysfunction in the world today (43 percent of women, 31 percent of men) is that, generally speaking, we were all taught that sex is about penetration. Many men have no idea how to make a clit sing, so women lose interest in having sex with them. A little dose of cliteracy could save a lot of marriages, you know what I'm saying?

Cliteracy Rule #3: She who owns the pussy holds the power.

Speaking of which, the world of healthy relationship is ruled by the woman's happiness, not her partner's. Why? Because when he prioritizes her, she makes sure that *he* is happy. If your pussy is not happy, the relationship is dead in the water. There's no game. We all know those relationships. We've been in them. We know there's nothing there, and yet the couple continues on, sometimes for years. Deeply unhappy with each other, suspended in relational formaldehyde. If you are in one of those relationships and you want to stay in it, you have only one choice: You must listen to pussy and call it out. You must change the circumstances and tell your partner the truth. If you don't, your partner will leave you, or you will die of boredom—or some combination of both.

It's pussy that both begins and ends relationships—not cock. Pussy *controls* the cock. She can get a guy hard across a crowded room, just by making eye contact. Try it as an experiment. Next time you see a man who turns you on, think about how yummy he is, and how juicy your pussy gets just by seeing him. Watch if he doesn't automatically come to attention. (By the way, there is no follow-through required with this research experiment. Sometimes it's fun to, ahem, erect a monument in your own honor—and then move on.)

When pussy is happy and turned on, a man responds by inviting her to go further and deeper. If she is unhappy and turned off, on the other hand, he will eventually go away. The only thing that makes a relationship work is a happy pussy. And the only one who can stand for your happy pussy is *you*. Your partner cannot read your mind. He/she cannot know what your pussy wants. You have to be the one to do the pleasure research and teach him/her the road map.

The reason my lover gets to stick around after all these years is because he knows how to pleasure me. He wants nothing more than to make me happy, and he continually up-levels his game to keep things fun and hot. I appreciate this so very deeply, and I give it back to him a thousandfold. But the only reason he does it is because my pussy is always happy to see him. Pussies that are fulfilled are exceedingly generous, and a woman's generosity is magnetic to a man.

Cliteracy Rule #4: She takes the time she takes—for very good reasons.

The elusive nature of female orgasm is an opportunity, not a problem. She takes her time because *there is no rush*. The sensual game for her is not about pregnancy or climax. It is about connection, intimacy, elevating her spiritual and emotional state, and fueling her life with pleasure. She is not there to get off, she is there to turn on and tune in.

The design of the clitoris, Natalie Angier writes, "encourage[s] its bearer to take control of her sexuality." Why? Because she works best when you treat her with love, honor, and respect. When you listen to what she wants. For our clits to sing, *we* have to sing. We can't lie there like Snow White, waiting for a prince to awaken us. Our clits are there to teach us that we are alive, vital, wildly sensual beings. We must step into learning our own instrument, so we can guide others how we like to play and be played. We have to learn the language of cliteracy in order to teach it to others. And once we have become women who can ask for what we want in bed, we can ask for what we want *anywhere*. Truly—bedroom to boardroom.

CLITERACY AND ORGASM

Cliteracy is about both the big picture and the very, very small picture. I'm referring, of course, to the locus of our 8,000 nerve endings. The centerpiece of our pussy; the grand dame of our pleasure: the clitoris. Understand, honor, and learn how to satisfy this sensitive spot, and you will create a bond of trust between you and your body that cannot be broken.

While the entirety of the clit is deliciously responsive, many years of research by the maestros at More University have revealed a single spot that is even more sensitive than the rest: the upper left quadrant. This sweet spot is so generous. It wants to feel more and more. Then, even more.

After two decades researching pleasure, I myself have clocked well over 10,000 hours of orgasmic practice. And my sensual training focused almost exclusively on that particular quadrant of my clitoris. When I started my sensual training, I considered myself orgasmic. What that meant to me was that I could have a climax—a fleeting but pleasurable "crotch sneeze." I was pretty happy with that. I didn't know that there was anything more available. Yet my sex life was not particularly transporting or nourishing. In truth, it was kind of furtive and confusing. Not that this bothered me; I had little idea of how important orgasm was.

Then I began my training at More, and in very structured sensual sessions I continually had my mind blown at the range and scope of the sensations I was capable of feeling. I flew like a butterfly, stung like a bee, soared like a shooting star, flowed like a river, poured with thick, gooey, oozing, honey-textured streams of sensation. I felt in my body what Kiri Te Kanawa must have felt singing "O Mio Babbino Caro." I saw God/Goddess. Felt my divinity. Howled with lust. Broke down sobbing at the beauty and wonder of my life, my body, the privilege of it all. Felt both the eternity and the ephemeral nature of being human.

The clitoris has limitless range of sensation, and limitless range of emotion.

Until I could feel this grandeur and expansiveness with my body, I could not live it within my small human frame. My divinity entered and inhabited me when I learned to come, and I could then fill out the brushstrokes on my canvas with the huge range of life that was mine to live. Coming made me the artist rather than the subject of my own life. The limitless nature of orgasm had me feel and know my own limitlessness.

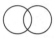

"GOING OVER" VS. ORGASM

There is a lot of confusion about what orgasm is.

Most of what we refer to as "having an orgasm" is a short ride to a high peak. There is a surge of sensation as you "go over" that peak. On the other side the clitoris becomes very sensitive—almost too sensitive to touch.

My sensual training focused on a different style of orgasm. I learned how to relax my body while my clitoris was stroked, and as a result I could experience peak after peak after peak with no "going over." In fact, the sensation would increase and expand to a point where it would even *exceed* the "going over" feeling. What's more, the sensation could continue for as long as I wanted. I quickly learned that this kind of orgasm actually *filled* my tank, rather than depleting it. I understood that my body had long been hungry for *orgasm*, not just "going over."

And as I discovered, what's good for pussy is good for woman as a whole. There is no upper limit to the amount of pleasure a woman is capable of feeling. The more she feels, the more she will want to make her partner feel. The more she is filled, the more generous she becomes. Living a cliterate, pleasurable, and pussified life is the equivalent of choosing to expand your range of sensation just like I did in my sensual training. In the end, listening to pussy teaches us how to take ourselves, and everyone around us, higher and higher.

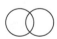

Most women in the world are operating from a huge amount of scarcity and ignorance in our sensual lives—and our lives overall. Women have been ignored for centuries. We were never the priority. Our hunger was never met. Instead of learning to feed ourselves, we have learned to ignore ourselves. Which comes with a huge price tag of rage, paid for by men and women in this world every day. Starvation makes for very poor manners.

That is why cliteracy is so important. The antidote to rage is not more rage. The antidote to rage is first shared grief, and then shared pleasure.

When I invite men into the School of Womanly Arts, I teach them everything they've longed to learn about women—and everything they have longed to learn about pussies. Once, one of my producers from *Late Night with Conan O'Brien* was in attendance. Some time later he told me he had called his mother after the class.

"Mom, why didn't you ever tell me about the clitoris?" he asked.

"You never asked," she answered.

This story has stayed with me for years because it so beautifully encapsulates the dilemma. The dilemma is that even if men *want* to learn about women's bodies and how to make women happy, we have no way of giving that information to them because our culture does not consider it important or necessary. We live in a world where men have no idea about what women really want, which is a great disadvantage. Women, for our part, have no idea that we hold the keys to the queendom. Imagine if girls grew up knowing that every part of their bodies—right down to the clitoris, whose only known biological raison d'être is pleasure—mattered? Imagine if boys grew up learning who women are, how our bodies function, and what makes us different from men? Oh, what a different world this would be.

Pussy is our true north, our meter reader, our highest power.

We don't trust her because we don't know her.

All that is about to change.

Grab a hand mirror and let's take a bit of a tour together.

A Guided Tour of Your Pussy

For the most part, we women know much more about a man's anatomy than we do about our own bodies. Straight women have spent way more time handling cock than we've spent handling pussy. (That includes our own.) As a result, most of us have been comparing our pussies to penises our whole lives and have found pussy coming up short. We've wondered what was wrong with her.

Why doesn't she turn on faster and get hard right away, like he does?

Why is she unpredictable and elusive, instead of the same every time?

Turns out we were right. *She is nothing like a penis.* She plays in a whole other neighborhood. And I want to give you a tour.

You can join in, if you want, or follow along with the illustration. If you want to join me, find a hand mirror and a private spot. Carefully disrobe, and use the mirror to gaze upon the unique and beautiful design of your pussy.

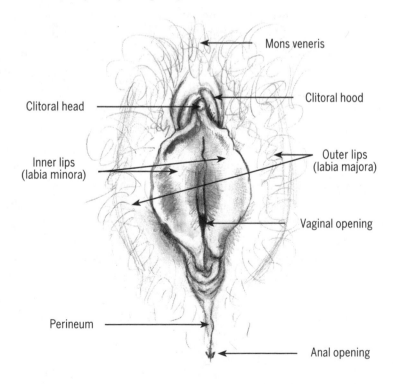

The first thing you will see is your *mons veneris,* or the "pubic mound." How do you know what that is? Look for its glossy, curly, delightful ground covering: your pubic hair. (Unless you shave or wax, in which case you will find less hair here—or none at all. But personally, I like a full bush. I am a woman, and I want to look like one. I don't like the porn industry dictating my fashion anyway.)

Your outer lips, or *labia majora,* will be covered in pubic hair as well. Not only does this pubic hair protect this important area, but it is so very receptive to sensation. Try this: Hold your hand a few centimeters above the lips. Notice the warmth, the energy, and the sensation of turn-on. Then lightly touch your pubic hair, and notice the sensation of turn-on grow. This is an important piece of information to begin to track. We not only want to know what our bits and pieces are *for,* but also how each one of them makes us *feel.* The more you know about your instrument, the more you can make her sing.

Did you know that this pussy you're looking at is a veritable ecosystem? Contrary to the Patriarchal World Culture's propaganda, pussy is totally self-cleansing. She does not need any outside or inside help to stay perfectly fresh and tidy. Moreover, every month—without being reminded—she ovulates and menstruates. Then she closes up shop, perfectly, with perfect timing, in menopause, continuing to cleanse herself through secretions from her vaginal walls.

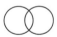

A WOMAN'S CYCLES

The cyclical nature of pussy is useful not just for reproduction, but also for tapping into your natural rhythms as a woman. For example, the three to five days before ovulation are an internal time. Your body's creativity turns inward. You'll probably have strong sensual desires during this period; you may or may not find yourself wanting to hump a doorknob. The five to seven days prior to menstruation is a more external, communicative time. In this window a woman is more likely to express what's troubling or bothering her. She might explode with rage, or with tears, or both. She will say what needs to be said. During ovulation, and again throughout menstruation, she just loves herself some carbs. A perfect meal would be truffle pizza, followed by spaghetti Bolognese, with ice cream and brownies for dessert. Rinse plates, repeat.

I once did an experiment for a few months, giving myself an orgasm every four hours during ovulation and menstruation. It reduced my food craving to next to nothing and dramatically eliminated my cramps. Why? Well, when we're in our "heat" cycle, the body is tumesced—swollen with sexual energy. This buildup of ungrounded sexual energy results in drastic and dramatic mood swings. We can be happy and loving one minute, irritated and angry the next. This roller-coaster ride occurs all the time in women, but is especially emphasized at that time of the month.

Tumescence is neither good nor bad; it's simply value-neutral energy. A cliterate woman will harness this energy and decide if she wants to embody it through orgasm, working out, cleaning the house, carb-loading, or yelling at someone. When she is aware of where she is in her monthly cycle, she can decide to use her tumescence in a happy, turned-on, pleasurable way. She can feel creative and productive and energized. But when a woman is not cliterate, she will disapprove of her cyclical nature and ignore her tumescence. As a result she may become irritated, angry, depressed, weepy, insecure, and/or lethargic. A cliterate woman never disapproves of her cyclical nature; she actually learns to use it to her advantage.

Menstruation was not always considered the huge bummer it is today. As Catherine Blackledge explains, in ancient Egypt people wore amulets of red stone that symbolized the menstrual blood of Isis, their most important goddess. The power of her blood was imparted to each person when they wore the red stone. In Calabria, Italy, a woman would save a few drops of her menstrual blood in a small bottle that she carried wherever she went. When she found a husband candidate, she would secretly give him a few drops of her blood in his food, and he would be forever bound to her. Sound crazy? What if you truly *were* that powerful?

Now let's continue our tour by getting a little more closely acquainted. Take your fingers and open your outer lips. If it feels more comfortable, use a bit of lube for this. You will see a lush landscape reveal itself. Her colors may astonish you. You may gasp and falter to find the words, like trying to describe a sunset to someone over the phone. Her color range can include the palest peach, the rosiest coral, the deepest red. She transitions from lavender to deep, dark purple, to milk chocolate, to dark chocolate, to rusty brown—and every color in between. All gorgeous, rich, delightful.

Your inner lips or *labia minora* can be found just inside the outer lips. Or, in some cases, peeking out from between the outer lips. Or, in some other cases, downright *protruding* from the outer lips. As Natalie Angier writes, the inner lips are "an exquisite origami of flesh." They vary in size, shape, texture—each woman's are gorgeous in their own way. Notice the glossy coating that adorns these lips. It is no accident; your lips are covered with sebaceous oil glands that produce a waxy substance called sebum. Sebum is not just pretty, it's also functional; it protects your pussy from infection and disease.

Gently use your fingers to open your inner lips. You will see your vaginal opening lying within. This is the cleanest opening on the body. She has a sweet, musky fragrance that is quite similar to a carton of fresh plain yogurt. This is no surprise, as your pussy's pH is the same as that of yogurt.

Run a finger lightly from the top of your vaginal opening straight north. At the end of this path you will encounter your clitoris. She may be easy to see, or she may be hiding under your clitoral hood. The clitoral hood protects this anatomical jewel, which as I've mentioned before is home to a whopping 8,000 nerve endings—all dedicated to pleasure. When the clitoris is in her natural resting state—meaning she is not sexually aroused—the hood covers her like a snug little blanket. When she becomes tumesced—sexually aroused—she engorges with blood. As she swells, the hood retracts. Suddenly she is open and ready for contact. Genius, isn't she?

The clitoris contains the highest concentration of nerve fibers anywhere on the human body. More than your fingertips, lips, or tongue. And you know how sensitive those parts are! Moreover she has twice the number of nerve endings as the head of a penis. Which explains why guys sometimes touch us twice as hard as we might like to be touched; they have nothing so sensitive on their entire bodies.

The clitoris is impractical. She does not "do" anything. A man's equivalent ejaculates, pees, and experiences pleasure. But your clitoris doesn't pee, menstruate, or ejaculate. She exists *purely* for pleasure. She does not atrophy after menopause. She will always be there for you, ready to connect you to the next pleasurable adventure.

When you look at her she may resemble a small bump. You may not be able to see her at all. Whatever she looks like, know that at most you're seeing her crown. The 8,000 nerve endings she contains actually extend down into our bodies where they cannot be seen. You can think of your clit like a wishbone; her crown is where the two halves of the wishbone come together. Then her shaft divides in two, with each root continuing deep into your vaginal canal. The famous G-spot is actually not a "spot" at all: it's part of the clitoral root that extends into the vagina. If you hook your finger inside your vagina and press in at the 12 o'clock, 3 o'clock, 6 o'clock, and 9 o'clock points, you'll feel different spots that are each pleasurable in their own special way. But the main attraction is still the clitoris.

LOCATION, LOCATION, LOCATION

The clitoris is the location of orgasm. Orgasm does not happen from stroking the inner or outer lips, nor the vaginal opening. All orgasm is cliterally centered. You cannot have an orgasm any other way. "Vaginal orgasms" are no exception—they result from stimulation of the clitoral root through the vaginal walls. When it comes to orgasm, it's all about the clit.

How close is the crown of your clit to your vaginal opening? Is she right there? Or a few centimeters above? The distance between the vaginal opening and your clit can vary by as much as an inch or more. If your clitoris is very close to your vaginal opening, it may be easier to have orgasms during intercourse. But if your clitoris is farther away, she will not have as much contact with your guy's cock when he penetrates you. In this case, your clit will require other kinds of attention and stimulation. Please note that only about 20 percent of women achieve orgasm through penetration alone. We at the SWA do not consider it a goal, so if you've been beating yourself up about not coming during intercourse, please let that one go.

Personally, my clit is not nestled up against my vaginal opening, a fact that in some way led me directly to the work I do today. As I mentioned in the last chapter, my first boyfriend and I spent a year playing around with each other's bodies before we ever had intercourse. Wow, that was a fun year! Then my boyfriend and I finally began to have intercourse—at which point I stopped him from doing anything but fucking me, because that's what I thought "sex" meant. Suddenly my interest in sex vaporized, only to be replaced by a disturbing feeling that something was terribly wrong with me.

As it turns out, this story is a common one. I hear it from my students all the time. How they feel "less than" because they have never come through penetration alone. Culturally we've been taught a model of orgasm that works for a man but not necessarily for a woman. Men's bodies work so differently than ours. A guy can get turned on at the sight of a woman, or the *thought* of the sight of a woman. He gets hard, and then he's ready to have sex. Most women are different. We warm up more slowly. We require more sensual attention before we want penetration. It's kind of like the difference between a cat and a dog. A puppy will run up to anyone and enjoy a good scratch. Cats take more time. They have to be seduced, studied. You have to learn how to approach carefully, and then how to make your pussy purr. Each pussy is unique, as is each woman. Good thing it is so fun to learn exactly how to engage with her! Paying attention to pussy is a pleasure in and of itself.

But we don't get taught about that. Instead, my students confide in me how they've questioned whether their partners are actually good in bed, or whether they themselves like sex at all. Fortunately, if you've ever had such thoughts, you're in good company. Marie Bonaparte, a colleague of Sigmund Freud, had the same questions. She researched female orgasm and concluded that women whose clitorises were more than 2.5 centimeters from the vaginal opening were "frigid." Frigidity was defined as an inability to have an orgasm during sex in the missionary position. Not wanting to be "inorgasmic" herself, Bonaparte actually had an operation to surgically move her clit closer to her vaginal opening—not once but *twice*. The "problem," however, was not resolved. So Bonaparte consulted with Freud, asking him to treat her for her problem. From the dialogue between them came Freud's famous quote, "The great question that has never been answered and which I have not yet been able to answer, despite my 30 years of research into the feminine soul, is 'What does a woman want?'"

This is a question that is ours to answer. Right here, right now.

Poor Freud had the question because we *women* do not even know what women want. I mean, look at us. Me, Marie Bonaparte, and billions of women throughout generations deciding there's something wrong with *us* because our bodies do not work like men's bodies!

I had disqualified myself from my own sex life at the tender age of 19 because I had learned that the way of men was *the* way.

After breaking up with my beautiful beau, who only ever wanted to make me happy, I did not know where to turn next. Was I gay? Bisexual? Asexual? I knew something was "wrong" with me, but I didn't know what. I decided I couldn't enter another relationship until I found out what was wrong.

It became my question. My quest. I didn't realize what I was looking for was cliteracy, and that I was going to have to write the book myself.

WHAT A WOMAN WANTS

So what does a woman want? Freud didn't know the answer, but then again he didn't have the benefit of talking to hundreds of women every year via the School of Womanly Arts. He didn't spend months interviewing women about their sex lives, their bodies, their pleasure. Lucky for you, I've had such opportunities, so I can answer this age-old question for you.

All things being equal, what women want is *orgasmic ecstasy.*

And then, after that, they want even *more* of it. More—and better.

More and better is never going to happen from the continuous use of the missionary position. Not for a woman, and consequently not for a man.

More and better can only happen from a repositioning and reprioritization of a culture so that the object of sex is not solely ejaculation or reproduction. When the objective of a sexual encounter between two people is sensual fulfillment, on the other hand, the whole game transforms. The positions change and the pleasure quotient expands exponentially and continually.

What's required is a level of confidence that only comes from cliteracy. Women who learn to relax into the pleasure our bodies were built to have also learn to trust themselves in a deep, cellular way. I am not talking strictly about sex here. Not necessarily. I am talking about *orgasmic pleasure.* I am not even talking about what we commonly think of as "orgasm," defined as "the physical and emotional sensation experienced at the peak of sexual excitation, usually resulting from stimulation of the sexual organ and usually accompanied in the male by ejaculation."

By the way, isn't it interesting—and telling—that in all the dictionary definitions of orgasm, the male orgasm is the one cited as representative, not the female?

Men climax very differently than women. They have something called a *venous plexus*, which is a tightly knit group of veins through which the blood enters and leaves the organ. During arousal, the muscles in the shaft compress the venous plexus, which means the blood can flow in but not out. Once a guy ejaculates, the muscles relax, the blood flows out, and his cock gets soft. Then there's a waiting period of around 20 minutes—the refractory period—that must pass before he can orgasm again.

The clit, for her part, has no venous plexus. Blood can flow freely in and out of the area, creating the potential for multiple orgasms with no refractory period required.

We grow up thinking that men are dedicated completely to sexual pleasure. But why, then, are we women the ones with an organ dedicated solely to pleasure? Men feel like they are king of the universe if they have three or four orgasms a night. Many women are capable of having *hundreds* of orgasms a night. (And if you're one of the women who can only have one, or two—you are perfectly perfect too.)

And how about the question of reproduction? Pregnancy requires some amount of ejaculation on his part, even if it's just pre-ejaculation. But for her, orgasm is not required for pregnancy. Doesn't it seem like some kind of design flaw?

Well, maybe yes. And maybe no.

Maybe the design of woman is trying to teach us something. Something wonderful and powerful about ourselves.

That each woman's *birthright* is pleasure.

That there need be no logical, practical reason for her to feel pleasure.

That she can, indeed *must*, have pleasure for pleasure's sake.

Sensual pleasure turns a woman on to her connection to her life force, her connection to her power. Orgasm teaches her to embody her true nature. It turns her on to feeling deeply, rather than scratching the surface of her connection to her life. She feels and enjoys the depth and breadth of her emotional instrument, both the laughter and the tears. She turns on her connection to *her* divinity (which she will never find in a church or temple), the part of her that is greater than her, the part of her that *knows*, that creates. Once she finds that divine connection, it allows her to move deeply from her own truth because she knows how to trust herself. She does not need someone outside of herself to give her a sense of her own rightness. A woman who is not turned on can feel swallowed or overwhelmed by her strong emotions. As she turns on, she begins to connect with her emotional instrument such that she is not victimized by her strong feelings but rather welcomes them as an aspect of her emotional range and power. Orgasm turns her on to her ability to know herself, her highest power, and her deepest truth—and stand for it.

No man can lead her to that awakening. Cliteracy is a road she must travel herself, in the company of her sisters. Women must teach other women about orgasmic potential. Because if we try to learn it from men—whose bodies are simply different from our own—we will not get very far. And "not very far" is where most women in the world are today.

A woman's sensuality requires her to take control of her pleasure. Her pleasure is sophisticated; it's not push-button. If she has control over her sexuality, and control and power over her decisions—for example, if she has sex with whom she wants, when she wants—she will have a good outcome. Her sex life will get better over time, and with experience. Great sex is all about attunement. It is about how attuned a woman is to her body, and how attuned her partner is to both her body and his or her own.

An important note: Pussy works best when her owner knows her. When she's been thoroughly explored, researched, and experienced by the one she serves. Pussy wants to spread her full wingspan in your honor. Women who have extended, massive orgasms in the bedroom, and who are in their fullest possible power in life, are women who have researched themselves. They've stroked their own pussies and have learned what feels good. If you ignore her—if you, yourself, don't ever touch her or stroke her or explore her—how can you expect her to fire up to full capacity when another is present? Without getting into contact with her, you might not even feel very orgasmic.

There are so many wonderful books on this subject; some of my favorites are *Extended Massive Orgasm* by Steve and Vera Bodansky, *Women's Anatomy of Arousal* by Sheri Winston, *Slow Sex* by Nicole Daedone, and *Woman: An Intimate Geography* by Natalie Angier. If you sit down and do all the exercises in these books for a month or so, you can make much progress toward expanding the intensity and duration of your orgasm. If you're feeling bold, you can even take classes in sensuality. See the Further Resources section at the end of the book for some suggestions.

There is also an incredible website—the best I have ever seen—called OMGYes (www.omgyes.com). This site was created by Lydia Daniller and Rob Perkins (along with a gang of tech geniuses), two friends who saw the absence of anything resembling a decent education about pussy on the web—and did something about it. It has a membership fee that is well worth the investment. The site hosts dozens of videos with women who demonstrate different techniques of how they like their pussies stroked. Perhaps the best feature is the interactive screen where you get to practice stroking and receive guidance on how to do it better.

I have taken incredible classes in Orgasmic Meditation by Nicole Daedone, who has a company called OneTaste. Also, sex expert Jaiya has amazing classes, private sessions, and a host of books and videos. Author Sheri Winston teaches great classes, and Layla Martin has a series of online programs that are excellent.

Thusly cliterate—that is, empowered with your own rightness, your own pleasure, your own orgasm—what is possible for you *outside* the bedroom? What is the spillover for a woman who knows her body intimately, knows exactly what she wants, and feels free and powerful enough to ask for it? This woman has inner swagger, outrageousness, and enthusiasm. Watch out, world. This is a woman who will bring her passion and fire to every aspect of her work and her life. Her voice will be heard, her opinions will matter, her points of view will be expressed. She will continue to drive the culture forward because of her deep connection with her own divinity. This woman is a role model for any woman who truly wants to live her legend.

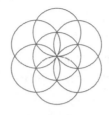

CHAPTER 5

THE WAY OF THE COURTESAN

It is not enough to conquer;
one must know how to seduce.

— VOLTAIRE

A few years after I had awakened my slumbering sensuality, I started a company called Relationship Technologies with my then husband, Bruce. We taught classes for both men and women, researching and exploring basic cliteracy. When I'd first encountered these teachings in my More University classes, they had changed my life. I wanted to give that same gift to other men and women, everywhere.

Not too long after we started teaching, I gave birth to my daughter, Maggie. To my amazement, my already-strong connection to the power of my pussy multiplied. Giving birth to Maggie was the most alive, joyful, and profound day of my life. I loved being pressed so deeply into the experience of my body's creative power. It was exciting, thrilling, expanding, ancient. I discovered myself to be more than I knew, more than I could have imagined.

I learned that my body *knew*. She knew how to create life, how to give birth, how to nourish this infant and make it happen. My brain was not in the lead that day; it was my pussy who ruled.

Holding my daughter in the days that followed, I noticed a deep sense of responsibility rising up inside of me. I felt the depth of my love and commitment to this brand-new girl, and as a consequence I felt a huge responsibility to the girls of today and the women of tomorrow. I wanted to help create a world that could handle who, and what, a woman truly *is*. Who could handle, and invite in, the Goddess I had first known when I was a child.

I needed to make sure I was doing my part.

I wanted to teach women to connect with their brilliance and power in the way I'd learned how to do. I wanted to help a woman turn on; to tune her inner pitch pipe to the key of her own irrefutable beauty and power.

My connection with my pussy had opened me to step more powerfully into this calling. I was no longer halted by my innate shyness, or my feelings of not being enough. I owned my pussy, and therefore I owned my life. I had no idea *how* I would impact the world of women, but I had no doubt in my mind that I *would*.

DISCOVERING THE COURTESAN

I got my first clue while I was breastfeeding—literally. Maggie was just a few weeks old, and I was doing my best to find a comfortable position to nurse her. The early days of breastfeeding were incredibly painful, but I was committed. To distract myself from the burning sensation, I turned on the television. Without realizing it, I had tuned in to a movie called *Dangerous Beauty*. In this period film, which is based on a true story, a young Venetian woman named Veronica is forced to give up the man she loves because her family has no money for a proper dowry. Veronica is given a choice: she can become a nun, or she can become a high-class prostitute (otherwise known as courtesan).

When Veronica realizes that all her hair will be cut off if she joins the convent, she somewhat unwillingly chooses the life of a courtesan. In the process she discovers that she has unexpectedly joined her own maternal lineage. Her mother had been a courtesan—an elite prostitute, catering to the 16th-century Venetian courts—just as *her* mother had been before her. As is the practice of the lineage, Veronica's mother begins to train her daughter in the ways of beauty and pleasure.

In one scene, as she is bathing Veronica, she speaks a line that went straight to my heart that day.

"If you want to give pleasure," Veronica's mother says, "you must *know* pleasure."

In that moment, it was as if a thousand lights turned on within me. I was brought back instantly to the night all those years before, when I had created a pleasurable experience for myself as a homework assignment for my sensuality class. *Dangerous Beauty* was reflecting back to me what I had discovered myself: that it is *pleasure* that connects a woman with her divinity and power. I was also discovering that this knowledge had once been handed down mother to daughter, in the lineage of none other than the courtesans.

I recognized that I, too, had been learning the ways of the courtesans through my sensuality training. I'd learned to *draw* pleasure from the simple acts of eating, bathing, walking, dressing. From allowing my gaze to connect with the gaze of a man. And, eventually, from touching his body. As I watched this mother teaching her daughter the art of taking pleasure from everything, I knew I wanted to be part of this lineage myself.

It had taken a very winding road, over the course of many years, for me to recognize that turning on and taking our pleasure is a sacred act for a woman. Yet during the time of the courtesan—the 17th through the 19th centuries, mostly in Italy, England, and France—it was a *known practice*. A courtesan was taught the art of pleasure because it made her more valuable; once connected to her power and divinity, she became irresistible. She became sacred; a direct conduit to the Great Pussy in the Sky. Yet this lineage, and its precious teachings, had been lost to modern women. With the advent of feminism, we were able to receive an education and join the workforce. But in the process of gaining the same rights as men, a huge part of our nature as *women* had been forgotten. Watching *Dangerous Beauty,* I recognized that the missing element in a woman's true education lay in pleasure and sensuality, and I saw what the lack of it was costing us. I realized that the reason women in B-school at Harvard could not raise their hands in class, or the women in Linda Babcock and Sara Laschever's book *Women Don't Ask* couldn't negotiate a fair salary for themselves was that they still stood in self-criticism and self-doubt rather than the free space of divine playfulness that the courtesan so beautifully modeled. I resolved to right that imbalance by starting a school for women. A courtesan academy for the modern world, where I would not teach women the *profession* of the courtesan, but her deeper legacy: the ancient art of being a woman. It is the stories of women leading a turned-on life that inspire us to do the same. Many women at my events find it hard at first to understand the difference between a courtesan and a prostitute. Like prostitutes, courtesans accepted money from men. Sometimes what they were paid for included sex, but just as often it included the pleasure of simply being in the courtesan's presence and receiving her inspiration. It was the role that courtesans played in society that differentiated them: they were the keepers of beauty, pleasure, and turn-on. In other words, they were the custodians of the sacred feminine. There is a huge difference between a prostitute—who fucked a man for cash—and a courtesan, who fucked a man back to life, or deliberately took him higher, or had a sacred spiritual sensual encounter with him so that he could connect to his soul again.

WELCOME TO THE SCHOOL OF WOMANLY ARTS

It was as if the courtesans of the past scooped me up and made me one of their own, as they will for you now. Books about the history of the courtesan lineage found their way into my hands, and I studied them carefully. I took notes on the ways of these living legends and began to enumerate, practice, and live their virtues. Virtues such as timing, beauty, cheek, brilliance, grace, and flirtation. Each courtesan's legendary story began with a powerful, very nearly overwhelming rupture, which she somehow flipped into an extraordinary opportunity for unimaginable greatness. I was going to do the same. In fact, I determined to be more than just a courtesan; I had the audacity to elect myself to the position of Chief Courtesan. I was responsible for training a world of women who were universally suffering temporary amnesia—having forgotten their beauty, their power, and their gloriousness. Having recently become a mother, I decided to call myself "Mama Gena." As headmistress of the courtesan academy, I would force women to have more pleasure than they ever dreamed possible. I knew I would have to push them ever-so-slightly against their will. No woman I knew—including myself—had grasped the vital importance of pleasure in a human being's life. My new school would be called Mama Gena's School of Womanly Arts. I held my very first class a few weeks after I first watched *Dangerous Beauty*, right there in my very own living room. I had just 12 students, but we were on our way.

I myself wanted to lean into the story lines I was reading and teaching, so I went about becoming a modern courtesan. Not by entering their profession, per se, but by enumerating their ways and practicing them in my own life. The courtesans were women who, during a time of almost unimaginable repression for women, did not fall victim to self-doubt and disempowerment. Because they were free to connect with their turn-on—both in terms of sex and in the broader world of pleasure—they were able to use the repression as an opportunity. To rise above it rather than succumb to it. In them I saw a new model of what a woman could be, for herself and for other women. In truth, this transition had already begun to happen to me.

For example, I discovered that the courtesans were capable of attracting everything they desired. I wanted to see if I could do the same. What would happen if I led with desire and attraction rather than practicalities or reason?

There was an ancient knowing that was reaching toward me, and I was paying attention. I was beginning to see that the courtesans played on an entirely different field, somewhere beyond the logical. I knew I had to shake off feeling small and insignificant. If I wanted to become a courtesan, I had to step up and become a personage. I chose to inhabit my radiance rather than my doubt. The courtesan had this inner gnosis; she knew that life is sacred. Thus empowered, she not only brought herself back to life but everyone she encountered.

Over the course of the next year of intense study, practice, and teaching, I discovered that there are some distinct "ways" of the courtesans. Some abilities they cultivated out of necessity, but which were rooted in the innate power of woman. I began to sketch these out for my students—an anatomy of the courtesan, but also of woman in general. Model yourself in the image of these remarkable women, I discovered, and get ready to watch your life transform from the inside out.

SHE ATTRACTS WHAT SHE DESIRES

What was the number one lesson the courtesans taught me? The power of desire. If there is something a woman wants, her desire alone is powerful enough to bring it to her. Of course, I wanted to experiment with this theory. I decided to allow my life to be driven by desire. In this lesson, I let Cleopatra be my teacher. Having been overthrown by her brother, she smuggled herself inside a rolled-up rug into the court of Julius Caesar. There she seduced the emperor and then convinced him to champion her cause: recapturing her rightful throne of Egypt. Her desire-driven story line has inspired us for more than 2,000 years.

Looking for a more contemporary role model, I found Sarah Bernhardt, who wanted to be a great actress. Herself the daughter of a courtesan, Bernhardt used her fervent desire to be adored internationally to create a fortune for herself—touring the world and living a most remarkable life of fame and adventure.

If these legendary women could do it, I thought, *so can I.*

The first thing I had to do was reach within. To follow my deepest desires, I had to know what they were. What I began to notice was that if I could *imagine* it, I could attract it. Seeing it in my mind's eye was enough to create something in my life. I started to think of desire as a technology, and I was constantly practicing how to make the most of it.

At the time I was reading *The Game of Life and How to Play It* by Florence Scovel Shinn. This small book, written almost 100 years ago, is all about how thoughts become things. Scovel Shinn suggests that if you dig your ditches and prepare the ground for the seeds, the seeds will be given "under grace and in perfect ways." Reading this book filled me with hope, which was something I very much needed because I was exploding with desires.

I wanted my little school for women to expand. I wanted to teach millions of women everywhere to access their turn-on; to step into the power that is theirs by divine right. I wanted to find out who Mama Gena was, and to have some fun with her. I wanted beautiful things—to live in a beautiful place and to write books and to travel. I wanted to be on television, teaching women about their magnificence. I wanted to be a spoken-word rock star and perform all over the world. I wanted to have celebrities and other movers and shakers as my friends. I wanted to build community and sisterhood, which I was discovering are the most important ingredients to a fulfilled and supported life. I wanted to create a beautiful home for myself and my family. I wanted romance and poetry and ecstatic sex and to live my own legend, whatever it was, just like the courtesans of old.

I had no idea how to do any of that, but I hoped the ancient knowing of the courtesans would teach me. I kept studying, paid attention, and began to follow their example whenever I could.

SHE DRESSES THE PART

Once Mama Gena was hatched, there came the question of what she should wear. I knew instinctively that I needed a signature outfit. Naturally I turned to the courtesans for inspiration. I knew that courtesans were distinguished by their fabulous clothes and jewelry. Charles Frederick Worth, a British clothing designer who had lived in Paris and was considered the father of haute couture, made clothes not only for the Empress Eugénie, but also for the most fabulous courtesans of his day. Like modern-day movie stars, the courtesans took the biggest fashion risks and allowed the designer to be at his most creative.

Poverty was no deterrent to the courtesans, which was good for me since I had no money. Courtesans were known for launching fashion trends with their incredibly unique and creative style, and they did it without the benefit of affluence. Each of them made the leap from poverty to fabulosity through wealth of an altogether different sort—so I began to look for it. One of my earliest finds was Émilienne d'Alençon, a famous courtesan of the belle epoque. Émilienne was blonde and rosy, and had created a perfectly cheeky and popular circus act at the Folies-Bergère. In the act she had a troupe of rabbits dyed pink, wearing ruffled paper dresses to match her own. I made note of her saucy humor and her intractable bravery. Another find was one of the greatest courtesans of all time, Marie Duplessis, on whose life *La Traviata* was based. At age 15 she was working as a milliner's assistant making wages that were too small to even keep her alive. But she was learning how to dress, how to do her hair, how to lose her country accent and speak perfect upper-class French. One day after work, she stood shivering and starving on the Pont Neuf, near a French fry stand, inhaling the fragrance. It was the middle of winter, and she had been hungry and cold for months. An average young woman might have been discouraged or angry or victimized by her impoverished circumstances. But not Marie. She stood on the bridge full of hope, full of desire, full of the anticipation of how wonderful one of those hot fried potatoes might taste. Wouldn't you know it: a gentleman crossing the bridge saw her and purchased a cone of fries for her. She wolfed them down with gusto, and when she looked up he was gone. A few years later, this same gentleman would encounter Marie at the Opera—this time exquisitely dressed and dripping in jewels, on the arm of Comte Edouard de Perregaux. She was a woman who was not afraid to be led by her enthusiasm, and who would not be stopped or discouraged by her humble circumstances.

These lessons in hand, I went to a thrift shop with my gay friend Pierre, who was an expert in thrifting. I had no money for a fabulous outfit, but I had the desire. Pierre had me try on everything in the store under $25. It didn't take very long for us to find the perfect pair of pink silk Chinese pajamas. Pink silk! Perfect for a courtesan. A store in SoHo had a matching pink feather fan for $10 and a boa for $5. It was so *Auntie Mame*! The outfit felt exactly right. The courtesans were teaching me the power of being unafraid to attract attention with my appearance. I wore that outfit for *every single class* I taught for the next year. I made public appearances in it. I posed for all my media in it. In the process, pink became the school color. Even though today I enjoy enough success to buy designer dresses for my live events—and have even had clothing designers offer to make clothes *for me*, for *free*—I still feel grateful for those pink pajamas. And I have been known to commemorate my humble beginnings by giving out pink boas at many live events that the SWA holds.

She Rises Above

Courtesans were not just kept women, they were *luminaries*. Personages. Dignitaries. They were cohorts to kings, emperors, regents, and statesmen. They were muses to artists, painters, writers, and sculptors. They were front-cover-of-*People*-magazine-worthy, the headliners in gossip columns, the sought-after subjects of great artists and writers. They were constantly arousing attention and adoration on the social circuit, foremost among the celebrities of their day.

Yet great courtesans were not born, they were self-made. The courtesan had to cultivate and develop herself. The ingredients that made a great courtesan were intelligence, profound self-awareness, a sense of outrageousness, a grand imagination, and turn-on to spare. But perhaps even more important, I discovered, was an unexpected ingredient: hardship.

A courtesan had to come from nothing. No advantages of birth, no money, no support, no rich relatives to fall back on, no opportunities. There is freedom when you know you're playing your only card. There were no other options for poor women; it was the convent or the courtesan. Discovering this thrilled and excited me. I had nothing either, so I fit right in. I loved knowing that "nothing" was an *advantage*. It forced the courtesan to shift her inner paradigm and turn the bitter landscape of her circumstances into a playground.

What I discovered, the more I entered their world, was that the courtesans saw their disadvantages differently than the rest of us. They saw their obstacles as a delicious *game*. I decided I was going to approach my dire financial situation as a game. Rather than charging a very small amount when I first started coaching, I decided to charge an audacious fee—and offer a money-back guarantee. I set myself up with the game of delivering results better than anyone (even I) could have imagined. It was terrifying and exciting, especially because the industry of coaching had just begun, and most of my clients had no idea what to expect. But each and every one of them had astonishing breakthroughs and results. I never had to make good on that money-back guarantee.

This move from victim to courtesan was the greatest spiritual backflip I had ever attempted. I'd heard of people who had valiantly *endured* troubles, which was, itself, a slight improvement over complaining about their trials and tribulations. (The latter being the way of my own heritage.) But to *profit* from hardship? To actually create living poetry from an impossible set of difficulties?

To greet the worst-case scenario as if it were a gift? Now *that* was interesting.

The courtesans were choosing to find the magnificence and radiance in their adventure, despite the circumstances. I had learned a similar choice in my sensual training. I remember once I was complaining that my partner was stroking my clit too hard. He stopped, but the teacher encouraged me to change my perspective. To *turn on* and choose to love the pressure of whatever stroke I was getting. To treat it as if it were the last stroke of my life. What I found was that I could actually *reinterpret the sensation* to feel incredibly pleasurable. I never knew I had that power. It was the same power I was now witnessing in the lives of the courtesans.

A courtesan believed utterly and completely in her own perfection, and that of her life. She charted her course with pleasure as her North Star. Joy was her compass. Even with all of my sensuality training up until that point, I had no idea turn-on could be *that* powerful.

SHE LIVES TURNED ON

To be sure, a courtesan's innate turn-on had to be met with an equal dose of curiosity and gumption. Starting from scratch—or far below scratch, in many cases—she had a huge learning curve ahead of her. She was meant to entertain the most elite men of the court, so she had to learn table manners and upper-class speech patterns. She had to learn to read and write, to play an instrument, and to speak articulately about literature and politics. The most extraordinary part was that these women had to accomplish all of this during a time when most women had no freedom, no right to own property or handle their own money, and no access to education. The courtesans had to turn a brand-new, almost unthinkable page, with almost no role models. As a result, they developed a secret knowledge that was shared among them: the art of being a woman.

This art allows a woman to defy her circumstances, rise above them, and create a whole new paradigm for herself. What is required is to combine the womanly virtues of grace, beauty, and charm with a level of brilliance and artistry that is powered by the ability to *turn on regardless of circumstance.* The courtesans infused themselves with the power of sensual fire, of life force. They were powered by pussy.

In her wonderful book *The Book of the Courtesans,* Susan Griffin describes a ravishing sculpture on the floor of the Musée d'Orsay called *Femme piqué par un serpent.* The model for this work, a courtesan named Apollonie Sabatier, is in an ecstatic swoon with a serpent. (Yes, it's a metaphor.) The famous poet Charles Baudelaire, similarly swept away by her charms, wrote this about Sabatier:

Your head, your mood, the way you move,
With a beauty like the beauty of the countryside,
As laughter plays across your face
Like fresh wind in a clear sky.

Sabatier inspired the besotted sound in Baudelaire's words, and the passion that the sculpture evokes, with the full force of her radiance. When a woman is turned on, she is in her highest power. She can capture a man with her gaze, her attention, her presence. A courtesan is a woman who is lit from within. She is plugged into her innate divinity. You can actually *see* when a woman is turned on or turned off. There is an inner light to her when she's turned on, which goes dark when she's turned off. Even if she is physically beautiful, she will not look radiant. Conversely, if she is plain or ordinary-looking—as many of the courtesans were—but turned on, her radiance illuminates her like a thousand inner candles.

Turn-on was the magic. It was the elixir that allowed courtesans to become fabulous. One dictionary definition of *fabulous* is "based upon or relating to a fable." A fable is a legend that inspires— literally *breathes life into.* With the telling of a fable, meaning is restored to life. The exquisite courtesan cocktail restored the meaning to life for everyone who encountered her. Every woman has the potential to be fabulous, to restore the meaning to life, for herself and others, when she plugs into her own eternal powers of radiant turn-on. I knew it was this experience I wanted to—*had* to—offer women through the School of Womanly Arts.

She Chooses Beauty

The courtesans loved, perhaps even worshipped, beauty. They required beautiful homes, beautiful jewels, beautiful dresses, and beautiful experiences. Just as every jewel is enhanced by a velvet cushion, these women seemed to understand instinctively that beauty translates to power.

Beauty was once considered sacred. In our culture today, it's presumed to be a passive virtue—an accident of good genetics. But not to the courtesans. More often than not, the courtesans themselves were not genetically beautiful. Rather, they *created* their beauty through considerable intention, determination, and skill.

I decided I could do that too. I had never considered myself beautiful, but I decided that I could change my mind. To help me choose to be beautiful, I studied women who had already made that decision. I began to watch women, like fashion icon Diana Vreeland, who was not a classic beauty but had impeccable posture and great style. When she spoke, you could not take your eyes off her. I studied the great movie actresses of the 1930s and '40s. I marveled at how an actress like Mae West, advanced in age and with a chubby body, found her way into films with dashing younger leading men—all of whom fell hopelessly in love with her. I would imitate the slower way these actresses walked, the way they took their time observing their features in the mirror, pleased by what they saw. The way they would hold a posture or a pose, as if waiting to be noticed.

I drew inspiration from how the Italian courtesan Nana was carefully and slowly groomed for her debut. She and her mother worked for months to draw out her beauty. Special creams were rubbed on her skin to enhance her coveted pale complexion. Her hair was placed over a large brimmed hat so she could sit out in the sun, lightening her hair while protecting her fair skin. In the same spirit, I began the habit of taking a bath every day, rather than a shower. I took my time putting on body lotion to keep my skin smooth. I developed a habit of looking in the mirror and winking at myself, which allowed me to practice a sense of confidence. I would read out loud a different poem each day, simply to inspire me.

Oh yes, I would choose beauty, inside and out.

If I was going to do something as culturally provocative as becoming Mama Gena, dedicating my life to teaching women to turn on, I decided I needed a beautiful brownstone in which to develop the school and curriculum. It just so happened that we were living in the basement level of one. Right around this time, the tenants who occupied the upper floors were moving out. It was the perfect space for the school—a triplex with room for our new baby girl and the business. It was also triple the rent we were paying—rent we were already barely able to scrape together each month. It was terrifying. Beguiling. Utterly illogical. But I was a courtesan, so I had to ask: What would a courtesan do? Would she be practical and wait until she could afford to move? No way. She would seize the day. Bruce and I put together every penny we had, along with a few handouts from cherished friends, a few dozen rolls of quarters, a wing and a prayer, to make the security deposit.

In my research about the ancient goddess traditions, I had learned that very often the worship of the feminine took place in caves. The opening of the cave was often painted, or even shaped, like a pussy. I decided that I needed to have the vestibule of the brownstone painted like a giant vulva. My friend and student Meryl Ranzer volunteered to paint it. The light on the top of the vestibule was the clitoris, and the walls were painted gorgeous pinks and purples and peaches and reds. We even put a coating of clear gloss at the top to simulate lubrication. Everyone who came in and out of the brownstone had the opportunity to make a wish inside the pussy. (Of course, whatever you wish for when you are inside a pussy will undoubtedly come true—something men have known since the dawn of time.)

Almost as soon as the last stroke on that pussy painting was complete, *The New York Times* sent over a reporter to write about what was happening at the school. After the article ran, the SWA took off like a racehorse out of the starting gate at Belmont. I was on the front page of *The New York Times* Style section, and I got a dozen book offers as a result. I was proving my theories on the courtesan with my very own story line.

She Elevates Herself

I knew, deep inside my cells, that this school was going to be huge. I might have been teaching classes of 12 women, but I knew that someday it would be hundreds, if not thousands. I knew the groundwork had to be laid and the stage set. I noticed that all headmistresses of elite institutions had something in common: each had a large portrait of herself hanging in the parlor. I decided that having a portrait painted of myself was the essential next move, stepping into my role as the headmistress of the courtesan academy.

One of my clients, Caroline, was a well-known portrait painter. I negotiated a trade of services with her—she would get an intensive coaching course with me, and I would get a portrait to hang over the fireplace in the brownstone.

It wasn't until the day before my sitting that I started to think about what I was going to wear. Glancing through my collection of mommy jeans and nursing tops, I started to panic. I called my best friend, Marcie, who didn't skip a beat. "We'll go to Bergdorf's," she announced. Now, I was this little hippie chick pretending to be the head of the courtesan academy. I'd never heard of Bergdorf Goodman, so I had no idea it was one of the most expensive boutiques in New York City. The next morning, Marcie guided me into the hallowed halls of Bergdorf's. I had never, ever seen anything so beautiful as this little jewel box of a department store.

Each item perfectly selected and perfectly displayed. The building itself was magnificent—all marble and chandeliers. It felt exactly as reverential and holy as I always wanted it to feel inside of a church. If they had charged admission I would have gladly paid.

Marcie found a salesperson who put me in a dressing room and began bringing in clothes by the armload. Marcie waved off the pants and blouses, and instead asked for evening gowns. The saleswoman came back with a Mary McFadden gown that was the most beautiful thing I had ever seen. The top was beaded in gold, teal, sea foam, cranberry, and silver, with a portrait neckline. The bottom was pleated silk Fortuny fabric, in a gorgeous combination of teal and sea-foam green. Alchemy happened the moment I zipped into that dress. I looked in the mirror and suddenly before me I saw Mama Gena. I *was* her. I saw my creation; I *was* my creation.

Then, I saw the price tag.

I was suddenly flushed, hot, inebriated. I felt the oxygen leave the dressing room. This dress was my ticket to everything I longed for, my ticket to being what I wanted to become.

And it cost $6,000.

And Bruce and I were barely making rent.

The moment the saleswoman stepped out of the dressing room, Marcie explained to me a custom of wealthy women. She said that rich ladies buy dresses, wear them once with the price tag on, and return them the next day. She told me this was a widely accepted practice, and I should not be embarrassed or feel bad. I could wear the dress to the sitting that afternoon, and then bring it back to the store tomorrow.

It was going to be more like checking a rare and precious book out of the library than actually making a purchase. I was still terrified, but I was resolved. I had to serve my radiance at all costs, and this dress transformed me. I was no longer the shy and introverted Regena. In this dress I was Mama Gena, the legend. I called Bruce to explain why there would be strange charges on two of our credit cards. (We had so little credit available, I had to split the charge.) To my surprise, Bruce didn't freak out too badly. I nervously clutched that $6,000 dress and carried it through the New

York City subway as I traveled downtown to the artist's studio. I sat still endlessly that afternoon, while Caroline quietly painted, but my mind was racing. Should I smile? Look imposing? How to be beautiful when I was so filled with angst? I didn't know. Hours passed. She painted. I stuffed Kleenex in my armpits to make sure I did not sweat in the dress. At the end of the very long day, she finally invited me to the other side of the canvas to see the painting. I was expecting to see a confection of sea-blue green and sequins.

Instead, I saw an outline of my face. The greenish-blue of my eyes.

She had not even begun to paint the dress.

I had no idea it took longer than one afternoon to have a portrait painted. Caroline was heading to Spain the next day. Our next sitting would not be for two weeks.

Before I could panic, Bruce called again. He'd thought it over, he said, and he thought we should keep the dress. If I really loved it and really wanted it, I should have it. He had no idea how we'd pay for it, but he wanted me to have it.

His gesture was romantic, foolish. But my experiment was about trusting the power of my appetite. Still, how could I agree to this? I had to call my friend Pierre for backup.

"Regena—you are not taking the dress back," he said immediately. "You are going to *step into the dress*. You are going to buy shoes for the dress, earrings for the dress, hose, and gorgeous lingerie. Next time you go for a sitting you are going to take a car service downtown, wearing the dress. You are going to learn how to get in and out of the car in a gown. Let the dress teach you how to be Mama Gena. Let the dress take you and introduce you to what you want to become."

I knew he was right. Like any good courtesan, I had to elevate my appearance, in order to elevate who I was in the world.

Like so many of the courtesans I read about, I bit off more than I could chew in those early years. Handling the monthly expenses of the brownstone, the $6,000 dress, preschool payments . . . it very nearly sunk me. My credit card was suspended.

I went on a payment plan for several years until the credit card company was all paid back, with interest. But the doors that opened for me were entirely worth the leap off the cliff with no net. As I always imagined, a number of years later the school became a glorious, fun, successful multimillion-dollar business. That is the fable-worthy power of a woman elevating herself against the odds. Taking a stand for our divinity—before any other values the PWC might want to instill in us—restores the meaning to life. It did so not only for me, but for the thousands of women who have been touched by the SWA. Inspiration is always worth the price of admission.

She Is Outrageous

The more I read about the courtesans, the more I realized they truly made their own rules. In a time when most women were slaves to societal conformity, this was the courtesan's genius. The women of this time had far less freedom than we have today. Women were never financially independent; they were always dependent on their husbands or fathers for money. A woman could not own property or make purchases on her own. Nor was she educated, except in the art of embroidery, singing, and piano. Her sole purpose was to attract a husband. Dependency was her chief asset.

The courtesans, on the other hand, enjoyed power, independence, and education. They had the ability to own property and to manage their own money. (It's no wonder that they eventually inspired the women's movement.) Given the cultural context of their time, their lives were truly outrageous.

One of my favorite stories is about two Parisian courtesans: Caroline "La Belle" Otero and Liane de Pougy. They had a friendly rivalry going over who was the most powerful, wealthy, and beautiful. There was an informal competition as to which of these beauties could outshine the other when they appeared in public.

Now you must understand, when a fabulous courtesan appeared in public, she stopped traffic. Everyone wanted to see what she was wearing. She created a gorgeous spectacle in her horse-drawn coach, clad in glorious gowns and endless jewels. The opera at the Palais Garnier in Paris was an especially fitting vehicle for a courtesan to display her magnificence. There was a huge staircase for entrances, leading to a fabulously ornate salon and terrace overlooking the city. Suitors had private boxes with separate doors that would accommodate a private tryst in the middle of the opera or ballet.

On this particular evening, Otero made her entrance, clad head-to-toe in diamonds, rubies, sapphires, and emeralds—layer upon glittering layer, from tiaras and necklaces to earrings, bracelets, and anklets. Not to mention rings on every finger! De Pougy entered next, the height of restraint—wearing only one simple diamond necklace. But not to be shown up by her rival, she had her maid following closely behind, carrying a giant stack of glittering jewels piled high on a red velvet pillow. She *wore* her understatement but was *followed* by her excess. The humor! The wit! The fun! So playful. I had never witnessed the like among women in my lifetime. It was not simply outrageousness for the sake of being outrageous—it was delicious, provocative, and celebratory. It honored each woman's power and place on the social stage of Paris.

Outrageousness is a side effect of a woman being in tune with her sensuality. A woman who owns her pussy owns her life. And when you own your life, you can take risks. You can have fun. You can be creative. So unlike women in our world today. It's heartbreaking to feel how little room for play there seems to be. We judge ourselves and criticize ourselves and find ourselves wrong *just for being women*. We are attacked and berated when we don't conform to a male standard. The courtesans broke through that wall, celebrating and honoring the feminine. They could do this because they understood firsthand the world's desire for it. Their appetites, their outrageousness, their magnificent and powerful desires made them who they were—and made them irresistible to the men around them.

Homework: Practicing Outrageousness

Following the lineage of the courtesan is an invitation for each of us to begin to celebrate ourselves in a bold new way. Outrageousness is like oxygen for a woman. To honor the legacy, I try to outdo myself with extravagant entrances at my live events. Last year I rode into a weekend program in Miami on a white horse with a Moroccan saddle. At a School of Womanly Arts weekend I might have a gang of hot men carry me in above their heads on a palanquin. Or perhaps I'll reenact my favorite rock star performing one of their greatest hits. It's all in good crazy fun.

What could you do, today, to celebrate yourself in a bold new way?

Wear every necklace in your jewelry box, instead of just one?

Wear your hottest dress or shoes to work?

Sneak your sexiest lingerie under your work clothes?

We have an exercise in Mastery, where each woman goes to the most expensive store in her neighborhood and tries on an extravagance. It might be a fur coat, some fabulous lingerie, a $400,000 diamond ring, or a $6,000 dress. The point of the exercise is not to actually buy anything; it's to press your edge to see what kind of lovely things light you up and make you feel radiant. The important thing is to learn what turns you on and cultivates your outrageousness. Why not try it today?

SHE USES PLEASURE AS HER COMPASS

I have often taken my advanced students to Paris. We go there to celebrate and honor the birthplace of the courtesan. Given all the stories I've read about its role in the lives of the Parisian courtesans, I wanted to make sure all of our advanced students had their chance to walk down the magnificent staircase at the Palais Garnier.

The first time I set foot in this building, my senses were overwhelmed with its beauty. It was as if the courtesans extended their magic forward and backward in time, welcoming me into their immortal playground. Awestruck, I climbed the elegant, curved staircase. Everywhere my eye traveled was another gorgeous sculpture tucked into a graceful alcove. The second floor was better than the first. I was swept away by the golden chandeliers, the intricately carved ornamental columns, the huge fireplace, the expansive—and very sensual—mural painted on the ceiling. I could almost feel my ball gown swish as I made my way oh-so-slowly across the floor. The place was built to inspire the most exquisite aspect of the feminine, which is her radiance.

On the second floor I saw dozens and dozens of narrow wooden doors, leading to private boxes in the balcony. I desperately wanted to go into a private box—to feel the red velvet chairs and see the opera house from the inside. Unfortunately, the day I was there the house was closed to visitors because there was a ballet rehearsal under way.

I felt a strange determination to see the inside of the house. A courtesan wasn't to be deterred merely because there was a rule against it! Desire was flooding my being. Looking for a way in, my friend Barb and I spied a couple of young custodians on the balcony floor. In very broken French, we explained that we would very much like to go into a box for a moment, to see the opera house. At first they said *non*, but we beguiled. We charmed. "Won't you show us, *s'il vous plaît*? *Juste un petit moment?*" They looked at us, and then at each other. With a conspiratorial smile, one of them told us to come back in five minutes.

Oui! Très bien!

Five minutes later, the two custodians—suddenly looking even younger and more attractive—ushered us through one of the narrow wooden doors. There we were, in a luxurious box, overlooking the stage. We watched, transfixed, as dozens of dancers leapt across the stage, preparing for the evening's show. It was a scene that had been immortalized on canvas by Degas, experienced in all of its opening-night splendor by dukes, duchesses, and kings. But as I knew from all my study, the secret stars of the scenes Degas painted were the courtesans.

The lineage of the courtesan must have been coming through me, because to my surprise one of the custodians guided me to a private part of the box. He took my face in his hands and kissed me, first gently, then more deeply. He leaned against me, and I could feel his hard cock against my thigh. In a moment of passion, he pressed me up against the wall—accidentally flipping on a light switch and briefly illuminating our box. The light triggered an alarm, alerting everyone to our whereabouts. The dancers came to a standstill on stage, while the guys, Barb, and I tore out of the private box. We plunged into the middle of a large German tour group, then carefully and quickly snuck ourselves out through the gift shop. The best part? Our two heroes somehow found us, followed us outside, and begged us to meet them later for a drink.

These guys were both young enough to be my sons. But what did it matter? I was covered in courtesan pixie dust, and when a courtesan is following her desire, she is eternally hot.

She Flirts as a Spiritual Practice

A favorite story of mine from Susan Griffin's book concerns a courtesan named Geneviève Lantelme, who was the favorite of a media tycoon named Alfred Edwards. Alfred's wife, Misia Sert, was understandably exceedingly jealous of her husband's mistress. Misia came to call one day to beg Geneviève to stop seeing her husband. She never got the chance. After having her butler frisk Misia for weapons, Geneviève overwhelmed her with her charm and hospitality. She asked if there was anything she could do for Misia. Caught off guard, the wife stammered something about her husband. Geneviève reassured her that she was not really interested in him, and she made Misia an offer. "My dear," she said, "you can have him back on three conditions. I want the pearl necklace you are wearing, one million francs—and you."

Misia immediately took off the necklace and handed it over, and said the million francs would be delivered to Geneviève's home in the next few days. The very moment Misia returned to her hotel, there was a package for her. It contained the necklace and a note, written on hot-pink paper.

"I have decided to forget the money and return the necklace," Geneviève wrote. "I am holding you only to the third condition."

Oh, I love this story so! It perfectly illustrates the transformative power of flirtation. Jealousy between a wife and a mistress is most often characterized by anger, bitterness, and desire for revenge. Emotions must have been running very, very high for both of them. Imagine the desperation and courage of Misia, coming to the home of her husband's mistress! Imagine Geneviève keeping her wits about her, even while angling for the position of wife herself!

This encounter could have gone badly for both were it not for the magnificently fun, ultra-powerful move made by Geneviève. In challenging Misia, she was doing so many things at once. She was inviting collaboration between sisters, with the gorgeous spell of turn-on as the meeting place between them. Sensual collaboration, as opposed to competition, is practically unheard of for women inside a patriarchal culture. In that moment, Geneviève recast Misia from an inferior and powerless woman begging to maintain her place, to an equal. With her spicy offer, Geneviève treated Misia as perfectly capable of getting everything she wanted. If there were such a thing as a woman throwing down the gauntlet for a game of thrust and parry, Geneviève had done it brilliantly. Misia could recast herself as a player rather than a loser. All she had to do was become willing to follow Geneviève's example: to throw the switch inside of her, and simply *turn on*.

From there, it was simply a question of desire. Who wanted Alfred the most? Might they like to share him? One thing we know for sure—the hottest pussy would win. She always does.

Flirtation is not only fun, it's also spiritually effective. If a woman is flirting, she is in her highest power. Nothing can take her down. She's living in a state of such delightful radiance that she can create fun with whatever comes her way. When we flirt, everything and everyone seems suddenly perfect. Most of the time we are not living that way. We're living in the state of right and wrong—which is pretty much the best that the PWC has to offer. But in flirtation, a woman sees life as an opportunity for expansion. Life is a game, where there are no winners or losers. Just different experiences, each designed by the deepest truth of all: desire. The magic elixir that fuels such radiant flirtation is her very own turn-on.

Flirtation is in a woman's DNA. Yes, that's right: You were born for it. It is one of the gifts of having 8,000 nerve endings dedicated to pleasure. Haven't you been captivated by a baby girl in a stroller, flirting with you in line at the supermarket? And who hasn't flirted like mad with someone's new puppy? Flirtation is nothing more than *enjoying ourselves*. Enjoying ourselves like the world is our playground. Enjoying life like we're kids at a carnival. Flirtation has no goal. Flirting with a goal is hustling. Hustling is not flirting, it's work. It's commerce. But when flirtation has no goal, we fall into the arms of our desires, without attachment. Which, it so happens, is actually the best (and only) way to get what we want. We're suddenly free to enjoy the gift of being a woman.

I was obsessed by flirtation. I could feel it was my superpower. Soon after the article appeared in the *Times*, I got invited onto *Late Night with Conan O'Brien*. I decided the only way I would be able to handle the pressure was to make sure I flirted from the moment I stepped into the studio to the moment I left. I knew the only thing that could mitigate my nerves was my own enjoyment. And I knew that the moment I started flirting was the moment I would become a superstar.

I also knew my desire was to become a regular guest on Conan—I wanted it with every fiber of my being.

They sent a town car to pick me up, which I enjoyed to the max. They gave me my own dressing room, filled with snacks and drinks and presents. There was no rehearsal—just a pep talk with the producer, who told me to stick to the topics we had agreed to talk about, and to *never, ever* ask Conan a question about his personal life.

I danced to the live music backstage. I winked at the guy who opens the curtain as I walked onstage in my borrowed dress and recently purchased very first pair of hot Prada pumps. I flirted and had fun with Conan. And at just the right moment, I played the most outrageous card—which is always the key to the courtesan's success: I broke the cardinal Conan rule. I asked him not just about his personal life, but about his *sex life*. Naturally, because I was so turned on, it drew a huge laugh and was a lot of fun for everyone—including Conan. That bold move cast me in the role of co-conspirator and player, rather than new kid on the block.

Over the next few years, I got my wish. I was invited back on the show six times, which is virtually unheard of. Most celebrities get invited once a year, when they have something to launch. I was invited back simply because Conan and I had fun together.

Studying the legacy of the courtesans had served me well.

She Never, Ever Gives Up on Her Desire

Perhaps the most powerful thing that the courtesans taught me was to never, ever give up on my desires. I was noticing that desires seem to have a life cycle of their own, and that it was very important to trust the timing of a deeply held desire. Timing, as they say, is everything. And courtesans had timing *down*. Coco Chanel is the perfect example. She was a courtesan, born in poverty in 1883. After she caught the eye of a wealthy protector, Étienne Balsan, a whole world was opened to her. As his mistress, she lived a life of luxury and social opportunity. Always independent and creative, she opened a hat shop and began designing hats.

A few years later, she met the love of her life, Boy Capel. He assisted her in opening her own couture shop in Paris. In choosing freedom and creative expression for herself, Chanel freed women from the bondage of corsets with her brilliant eye for fashion. Her timing could not have been better. She reached for the world and the world of women's fashion reached back, and continues to do so. The power of Chanel's desire was so strong that her signature look—string of pearls, quilted bag, tweed suit, little black dress—still have incredible power among the fashion elite.

When Chanel started her business, she simply made hats. It took years for her to find her footing and establish herself as an über-successful international brand. She started by using the sewing skills she'd acquired in her early years in the convent—and she did not stop until she was the most successful female entrepreneur in the world.

I began to see—and trust—that the Great Pussy in the Sky had my back. She was conspiring with me, and with all women, to make sure we got to live our dreams in our lifetimes. It was my mission to connect women with their most deeply held desires. My job was to fan the flames of women's desires and to make sure they were paying attention to what they wanted in order to create (or conjure) it.

Never, ever, *ever* giving up on a desire is both easier and more complex than any other move the courtesan makes. Easier, because you simply locate what you want and enjoy the thought of having it—regardless of how long it takes to acquire it. You enjoy the pleasure of wanting, rather than disapproving of the fact that you do not have it yet. Feeling turned on at the thought of a desire actually sends an energetic vortex of attraction out into the world. Everything in your world begins to line up around that desire. The way to shut down the vortex is to disapprove of the fact that you don't have it yet, or to doubt that you'll ever get it. Indulging in doubt is throwing water on the fire of desire.

As for the complexity? When we open ourselves to desire, we open ourselves to being completely remade. A desire is the interface between you and that which is greater than you. Every woman is a legend, with her lid on. But a legend with a lid is a legend that never gets to live. Every woman's legend must be *lived* in order to feed the evolution of the world.

We will never live our legend if we follow someone else's script or someone else's road map. Listening to and living our desires as if they were a road map to our truth is the way we women live our unique, phenomenal gifts. Each of us has a unique voice that the world requires. And the key to unlocking this gift is to cherish your own story line and to stand, with every fiber of your being, for the significant and momentous importance of your desires. Everything you want *matters*. It matters deeply—not just to you, but to everyone. We are all impacted, influenced, and shaped for the better by the radiant power of a woman's desire.

It's terrifying to surrender, and terrifying to become greater. Far more terrifying than staying small. It is the ultimate hair-raising adventure to toss your saddle astride the unknown and gallop in the direction of your desire. But there is no more spiritually alive way to live.

When I was divorcing Bruce, I decided that I had to return the engagement ring that he had given to me. My divorce attorney disagreed with me. He knew that I had no money, and he thought I could easily get a few thousand dollars for the ring. But I was not deterred. I pressed the ring into my lawyer's hand and told him I had to return it to Bruce because I was making a space for legendary love in my life. I wanted to leave a space for a man who truly saw me and truly loved me for everything I was. I wanted *that* man to put a ring on my finger. I knew if I kept the engagement ring, I would never be fully open to something even more wonderful.

What I did not understand at the time was that becoming a courtesan—and plighting troth with my desires—in no way guarantees a fairy-tale ending. Desire wants what she wants, and sometimes we have to be taken apart in order to be put back together in her image. I did open the space for legendary love. And in doing so, I opened the space for an experience more harrowing than I'd ever gone through, or could even have imagined. I opened the space for devastating *rupture*—which is a place every woman must go, if she wants to become the woman she is meant to be.

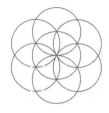

CHAPTER 6

RUPTURE

Doubt thou the stars are fire;
Doubt that the sun doth move;
Doubt truth to be a liar;
But never doubt I love.

— Hamlet's letter to Ophelia

Living one's desire is an adventure like no other. There are no safety nets, no seat belts. In fact, when you plight your troth to your desires, you're kind of asking for it. You're grabbing the hand of the Great Pussy in the Sky and asking to be *broken open*. Asking to be *remade*. Asking for the current version of you to be *shattered and reassembled* into the woman you were born to become. This is part of the life cycle of what it means to be a woman. Just as the seasons are cyclical, with winter as necessary as spring, and the sun and moon move in cycles, with times of light and times of darkness, so moves the body and soul of a woman. We each require the dark night of the soul as much as we require the light.

The word I use to describe this undoing? *Rupture.*

Rupture comes from the Old Latin word *rumpere*, which means "to break." And broken is exactly how we feel when we rupture. It might be the result of a devastating loss: a divorce, the death of a loved one, or the loss of a job. It might come through some catastrophe—a war, a fire, a rape, a flood, an illness. Oddly enough, we can rupture just as easily when something wonderful throws our lives into chaos—like giving birth to twins, relocating for a new promotion, or getting cast as the lead in a Broadway play.

Rupture is a natural part of life, and a natural consequence of desire. For whenever we get something we want, we must say good-bye to what we had. No matter how dissatisfying it might have been, it was familiar. Perhaps you desire a relationship, for example. When you finally meet someone and fall in love, your life as a single person must end. Just because you've gotten what you wanted doesn't mean you're going to feel uncomplicated joy. There will be a sense of loss as your former life disappears before your eyes. To move ahead as the happy half of a happy couple, you'll need to mourn, even briefly, the world of being single.

But in the world of the PWC, we women have lost the sacred art of rupture. We've spent our whole lives trying to look good; trying not to show our strong emotions; trying to hold it all together regardless of the natural forces trying to take us to pieces. We don't want anyone to see our dark side, or to know how intensely we feel. We believe that our passion is wrong and that our deep emotions will only upset people. So we try to hide those feelings by stuffing them inside. The consequence of this is that we never really trust our own feelings, and we never really want to risk living our most deeply held desires. We opt to stay safe—to live the PWC version of ourselves—rather than risk being the gorgeous, bloody, raw, lusty, greedy, emotional, and appetitious creatures we actually are.

I myself learned about rupture in a very dramatic way. For—no surprise here—my *desire* was very dramatic.

I wanted nothing other than a legendary love.

Not just a regular vanilla love—I wanted *legendary*.

I had a child. I had a brownstone in New York City. I was Chief Courtesan at the School of Womanly Arts. I had everything a woman could ask for. Except that Bruce and I had divorced, and I was ready to *really love*. That was all I wanted. A love that was legendary. I had dreamed about it for years, as I'd never felt a true soul connection in my marriage.

I thought I was up for whatever it took to have that experience. Little did I know that my desire was setting me up for the greatest rupture of my life.

Legendary Love

Some people you meet. Not Dr. Tiitus Siegmar. This man, I *encountered*.

I first laid eyes on him at an art opening. I was still married at the time, and my daughter was a baby. From the moment we were introduced, I knew I was talking to the grandest man I had ever met. He was an art collector, a philanthropist, a venture capitalist, a genius, a huge player on the world's stage. So it came as a complete surprise to me that he actually seemed interested in the work I was doing. He seemed to find me, and the fledgling School of Womanly Arts, to be *significant*. I did not feel as important as he seemed to believe I was. But secretly I hoped he was right.

Over the next few years, Tiitus would call occasionally with an invitation to some philanthropic event or dinner party or whatever. His face always lit up when I walked into the room. Even though we were not yet all-the-way good friends, he would pick me up and twirl me around like I was a little fairy. I was in awe of him and the huge scale on which he lived his life. He was European. He walked fearlessly in the world of investments and economics. Yet he moved and spoke slowly, deliberately. He served on several museum boards, was a generous patron of the arts, and read about 30 books at a time. He conducted himself as if he were a king, always surrounding himself with simple but extravagant beauty. His 10,000-square-foot loft was filled with enormous works of art—a collection so vast he had to rotate it every six months to make use of it all. He would invite me to huge formal dinners for 40 guests, all of whom seemed to have won a Nobel or a Pulitzer.

Physically, he was a huge man. Well over six feet tall and heavyset, with gorgeous blue eyes. But inside, his soul was so gentle. So sweet. I immediately saw past the great man to the lost lonely boy within, and I felt somehow protective of him.

But he scared me, too, because he was so accomplished and so successful and so brilliant.

After Bruce and I separated, Tiitus was the first person to ask me out. As a newly single woman, my circuits were exploding. I had never thought of Tiitus as a *date*. I thought of him as a Great Man. Far too awesome and accomplished for me to even consider as a lover or boyfriend. But when he called, violins played inside me.

My *lady* came out to play with this man. The lady who could afford to take her hand off the wheel and surrender to being driven. The lady who was coiffed and cared for and generous with others. All this happened inside me when I heard his voice. He made space for a part of me no man had seen before.

Dining with Tiitus was an adventure. He believed utterly in great food and wine, and great art. There was no expense spared. We drank Domaine de la Romanée-Conti Montrachet Grand Cru with the appetizer course, and 1961 Château Margaux with the entrée. When the meal was finished, there were always two town cars waiting, one for him and one for me, and I was whisked safely home. Very sexy.

He and I lived in two different worlds. He was upscale and I was scraping by. A month or so after our first date, he asked if I wanted the keys to his Southampton estate for the weekend. To me, this was an overwhelming offer. I was still wobbling from the impact of my divorce the year before, struggling to find my footing. He knew I was a single mom, but he had no idea the financial straits I was in. I was less than broke. I had been unconscious around money when I was married to Bruce, and I had no idea we had not been paying our taxes. When we divorced, I received full custody of our daughter—and full custody of a $250,000 tax debt. I was determined to pay back every penny, and support and raise my girl in a beautiful way. I had no idea how I would do this;

I only knew that somehow, some way, I would. To be offered a weekend respite was just what I needed.

I had never been to Southampton. I had no idea how gorgeous it was, how luxurious, how exclusive, how expensive. Tiitus's house, which he rented from the Roy Lichtenstein estate, was a beautifully decorated "cottage" with acres of gorgeous landscaping, a pool, and a private pathway to the beach cut through the center of a privet hedge. I had never even *imagined* a place of this majesty and luxury and beauty.

While wandering around the gorgeous home, I found myself looking through his music collection. I noticed that all the music he had was tragic. Édith Piaf. Billie Holiday. Italian opera. I wondered why this great man would choose only heartbreak. Seeing someone's music collection is seeing into their soul. I was taking him in at a new level. He was majesty, heartbreak, luxury, generosity, and huge grand space.

When I was a little girl, I played with a box of handmade dolls under my bed. I took these dolls on grand adventures, rescued them from danger, gave them sensual awakenings, followed their royal journeys. I had rediscovered this box of dolls from my childhood after I met Tiitus, as a result of a conversation with him. He said that the things we played with as children are art. I was touched and astonished at how he inspired me to value this sacred bundle. Opening it, I was beyond surprised to see that each doll looked like someone in my life. There was one for my ex-husband, one for my daughter, a handful of close friends, and . . . Tiitus. I realized that the imaginary games I had played as a little girl were not games at all. They were desires that were now coming true all around me. I took it as a sign from the Great Pussy in the Sky. Perhaps the reason Tiitus was in my special box was because he was supposed to be my destiny—my legendary love.

Being in his house, feeling his generosity, sleeping in his bed, my toothbrush placed next to his, I was flooded with one word.

Yes.

Yes to Tiitus. Yes to this house. Yes to this man, to this adventure. Yes to the music collection, yes to Southampton, yes to his shy smile, yes to the way I already loved him. Yes, I would make him mine. Yes, he was already mine. I felt that this was the Great Pussy in the Sky giving me a chance at that for which I had always longed: legendary love with a great man.

When I was growing up, we had a housekeeper named Wilma who raised me. She would tell me stories about her life in Virginia, where she'd picked tobacco from the time she was eight years old. She told me her husband had been stolen away from her by a woman who had put some of her menstrual blood in his food. This story lurked in my imagination for years; it seemed to reinforce all I had learned about the power of pussy. This story smacked of real power. The kind you cannot mess with.

I decided to reach back in time and call upon the irrevocable power of pussy—and all my ancestresses from ancient Egypt to 20th-century Virginia—to ceremonially stake my claim. I walked around Tiitus's house and placed a drop of my pussy juice on every object in it, including his toothbrush. The rest of the weekend, I was not a guest. I was the lady of the manor.

The Indecent Proposal

Over dinner a few weeks later, I propositioned him.

"Tiitus, you and I have been friends for a long time, haven't we?"

"Yes, Regena."

"I have been thinking about us. It is time we became lovers."

He dropped his fork.

Then, he paused.

Finally, he looked me in the eyes as a smile spread across his face. "Very well, Regena. Agreed. Wonderful!"

He thought it might be nice to take me to St. Bart's for a weekend, take two hotel rooms, and get to know each other. I loved this idea.

But he never called.

I finally called him and got sent to voice mail. Over and over. I was crushed. A month passed, then two. I ran the gamut of emotions. Furious, frustrated. I hated him one minute, worried about his well-being the next. I finally left him a message saying that it would have been nice if he just told me he had changed his mind about us.

With this, he called back. Apologized. Explained. He'd had a serious health scare: a melanoma had to be removed from his back. He had not wanted me to worry.

Over the next few weeks, we skipped dating and plunged right into deep connection. I saw him through the health crisis, sat by his side at Sloan Kettering, met every doctor with him until he emerged from the surgery cancer-free. I felt honored—even privileged—to be by his side.

A few weeks later, at dinner at the Four Seasons, I told him I was very much in love with him. That I believed our relationship was destiny. That night, instead of two cars coming to drive us home from dinner, there was one. We kissed for the first time in the backseat of the limo on the way home.

The experience of being with Tiitus was like nothing I'd ever known. It was like there was him, there was me, and then there was this third entity, which was *us*. I had never had an experience of *us ness* like that. It was tangible. It felt like a place in time and space—a beautiful place. Like standing in a meteor shower at night, darkness all around, stars above, and this blast of sparkling light showering over me. If it were music, it would be an opera. A symphony. With slow movements, passionate arias, crashing cymbals, tender strings. If it were poetry—what am I saying? It *was* poetry. I had gotten myself my heart's desire: a legendary love. I was no longer hoping for it, longing for it, wishing, waiting. I was in it.

A few weeks later, Tiitus took me shopping for my birthday present. We went to a jewelry store on Main Street in Southampton, where we saw a ring with a gorgeous, fat pink tourmaline surrounded by diamonds. He said, *"That* looks like Mama Gena. Do you like it, darling?"

"Yes," I whispered. "I love it."

"Wrap it up," he announced to the clerk, not even looking at the hefty price tag. I was overwhelmed. Not just because he'd bought me an unimaginably beautiful ring, not just because he was by my side, loving me, not just because I was living this dream. The ring I had promised myself would come to me after my divorce was now on my finger. Placed there by a man who loved me, and who I loved in return.

I had never, ever been this much in love. I had never felt so guided by the GPS to my destiny.

Previously I'd always felt desperate in relationships. Or lost, or trapped, or striving. Or forcing the issue. Or helpless. Or clueless. This was a different feeling. It felt calm, exciting, relaxed, sexy, smart, intellectually challenging, safe, vast. Part eternity, part right now. Glamorous and simple. Fresh, healthy. Bracing, like fresh lemons. Thirst-quenching, like water.

I was so fucking grateful for this.

THE CRASH

I was at Tiitus's house in the Hamptons with a group of my girlfriends. We were having a really fun weekend, despite my disappointment: Tiitus was supposed to be with us, but he'd had to fly suddenly to L.A. for business. We went to the beach anyway, and then took an S Factor pole-dancing class—an amazing practice I'd discovered that gave women of all ages, shapes, and sizes a whole new way to embody their feminine. Storming out of class at 9 P.M., we decided we needed a piña colada and some cigarettes. We were pulling into a gas station to acquire the cigarettes when the phone rang. It was Tiitus. I picked up and immediately accused him of calling just to find out how my sexy dance class went.

He was quiet. Perhaps I was not in a place to handle some serious news?

Of course I was available, I said, the blood draining out of me.

It was his 30-year-old son, Niklas. He had been playing beach volleyball in L.A. and gone for a quick dip in the ocean. He dove into the water and hit a sandbar. His neck was broken. He was being taken to the hospital and Tiitus was on his way there.

As soon as I put down the phone, I realized I had to go to him.

My friends drove us home immediately. I organized childcare, made a plan for the week at the office, and prepared to go. As my friends packed, my daughter, Maggie, got in the shower with me and we had a knock-down, sobbing good-bye.

The first few days in L.A. were incredible. Incredibly hard, yes, but we had our teamwork well in place, having handled Tiitus's medical emergency together. But as the days turned into weeks, things began to disintegrate between us. Tiitus did not want me to come with him to the hospital anymore. He said I was too radiant and happy. He told me that his ex-wife and Niklas's fiancée, Jackie, did not like having me around. So all I did was wait for him at the hotel, doing my best to support him in any way I could. He seemed to be always angry and irritated and distracted, as anyone in his position would have been. All he cared about was Niklas getting well. He had no space for me.

I understood completely, yet my heart was broken. Only a few weeks prior, I had been the center of his world. Now I wasn't even invited to help. It was time for me to go back to New York. To leave my love and return to my daughter and my company.

My father died a few weeks later, after 10 years of slow decline into dementia. I could barely feel that loss, so overcome I was at the loss of my fairy-tale dream life with Tiitus. He would communicate with me for a bit, rage at me, then cut me off. I understood that he was a man in unimaginable heartbreak, and yet I could not stop myself from feeling furious and devastated.

I was angry at the Great Pussy in the Sky for shining her light on me and then cutting me off so heartlessly.

By the spring there were small signs of reconnection, but it was different. When we'd begun dating, I had felt like a teenager, barely touching the ground. Overwhelmed by him, his house, his wealth. By the fact that he was actually interested in me. Now I felt my heart in the aching verse of Puccini, of *Tosca*. Our life was a movie, and the soundtrack was the music that filled Tiitus's music collection. Tragedy. Heartache. Loss. Even when he held me, or cooked dinner for me, I could tell his thoughts were elsewhere.

Over the next year, I continued to reach for him, and he pulled away. He lived mostly in Los Angeles, I in New York. We saw each other once in a while, but he was absorbed totally in Niklas's recovery. I was frustrated and angry one second, desperately grateful to see him the next. I wanted my love to heal him; I wanted us to find salvation in each other's arms. But some door had shut inside of him. I couldn't get through, couldn't get in. I didn't understand but I wouldn't stop trying.

Then, it was over.

I was in Las Vegas with my best friends when I got the phone call. Tiitus was supposed to have been with me on that trip, but he had backed out at the last minute. The call was from his housekeeper, Lily.

Tiitus was dead.

I howled like a wild animal.

Dead? I could not process it. I couldn't do anything but weep.

This rupture was total.

I somehow made it through the next few days. I flew to the memorial service in L.A. and cried harder than anyone there. I talked to Tiitus's doctor. I had to know the sequence of things. When did he know he was dying? The doctor said that Tiitus knew the melanoma had returned the previous year, but he had not returned for further treatment. No chemotherapy. No radiation. He wanted to go on his own terms.

So Tiitus had known. He had not wanted to drag me down with him. He was protecting me by pushing me away in the last few months.

It was not that he didn't love me. It was that he *did.*

RUPTURE

Grief had overtaken my body, my heart, my soul.

I could not move in this grief. I could not leave this grief. I did not know who I was, nor why the Great Pussy in the Sky had forsaken me. I had never experienced anything like this before. I had been brought to my knees by divorce; had broken up with lovers; had lost a late-term pregnancy. I thought I knew tragedy and devastation. But this experience took me down to a depth of despair I had never encountered. The little girl in me who had been abused had found safety in Tiitus's arms. The courtesan in me had found inspiration in his bed. The struggling artist in me had felt a safety net in his wealth. The single mother in me had tasted the potential for partnership with our children. I'd thought he was the reward for all the hurt, all the pain, all the struggles I'd been through. I thought that meeting him and loving him was going to be my happily ever after. He was my legendary love; all that I had been striving for and longing for. The man in whose arms I found home.

I hadn't had a clue what rupture was before Tiitus died. I had never been so utterly decked, so cut off, so betrayed by my Goddess. How could the GPS do this to me? I was enraged one second, collapsed in grief the next, railing at the stars the next. What was I to do with this legendary love—whose story did not turn out as I had imagined?

My mind knew this love was over, but my body was taking her time. She was like my slow little sister. Still turning and yearning when we had to pass through his neighborhood. Still feeling stabbing pain at the thought of his death. Hardly breathing when certain songs came on the airwaves.

Some part of me did not want to move forward. Not yet. I surrendered my direction to follow hers. She had things to teach me that exterminated my will. She did not give a shit about deadlines or proper mourning periods. She wanted to sit on the ground and cry until she was finished.

It was a luxury I'd never had as a child.

I had never cried. Never cried when I was beaten by my brother. Never cried when I was sexually assaulted as a teenager. Never.

But now, I cried. I let my body guide me.

The grief was so big, there was no fighting it—only listening. So I listened. To *her*. My devastated little body.

She wanted this grief to move through her, physically, several times a day. So I let her have that. I danced. I wept. I moved her hips, her breasts. I arched her back, I twirled her around a dancing pole in my S Factor class, weeping.

She wanted massages. I complied.

She wanted to wear black velvet. Black anything.

She took me where I'd always been afraid to go: to the raging, grieving heartache that no one saw. She picked up where I had abandoned her, oh-so-many years earlier. When I was a child, there were no safe arms to crawl into, no places to feel what I felt. So I sucked up the pain and stuffed it inside, trying to do my best to stay strong. That's how the PWC wants us to be, like PWC-approved men: predictable, solid, and disconnected from our feelings.

But here—in the midst of this unimaginable loss—is where I found it. The gift in the rupture. *Rupture's gift is the chance to feel the pain that we could not afford to feel before.*

In rupture, this pain becomes *ours*.

Because we have longed. Because we have loved.

Tiitus had been the answer to my body's yearning prayer. I had thought my yearning was the love of this man. But what I got was an experience of pain so great that it reconnected me with myself. It reconnected me with every woman in the world who has been brought to her knees by devastation. And then, eventually, it reconnected me to the native wisdom of the feminine. It taught me how to be remade into the woman I was meant to be.

I thought I was in Tiitus's life to lift him from his suffering into my radiance. But it was actually the other way around. *I was in his life so he could break me apart and teach me to taste and touch and experience and own my darkness.*

RADIANCE IN DEVASTATION

The next month I was back in the Mastery classroom. I told the story of Tiitus and me. My students had been with me throughout the whole love affair. I had written the first season of Mastery in Tiitus's arms, in his house in Southampton, in the hammock in his yard. So there was no hiding what was happening inside of me. I had created a devastation that was so big, so vast, that it had broken me. I thought that my legendary love would rescue me from all the hardships and difficulties of my life. What I actually needed to learn was how to rescue myself. I needed the full weight of our relationship and his death to blow up all of my girlhood dreams so I could finally grow into the woman I am today.

Today I thank the Goddess for setting things up so well.

Without a loss of this magnitude, I never would have understood the reason I had been fighting like an unstoppable guerrilla warrior to set the School of Womanly Arts on its feet. I was giving my heart and soul to make sure women could connect to their power, their voices, and their radiance in this lifetime. I was doing it because of my own inability to connect to *mine*.

It was only because of the enormity of this experience that I was able to make the connection between the journey of a radiant woman and that of the courtesan. It was through my grief that I mapped out the journey of our courtesan lineage—the journey of being broken and remade, over and over, throughout the course of a lifetime.

In the hand of the courtesan I found the key to unlocking the spiral of my rupture, my grief. The key was her willingness to be the author of her own story.

The author, rather than the victim.

No matter how big, how grand, how deep the devastation.

Because she was plugged into her turn-on, she became the creatrix of every step of her adventure.

We all know women who blame their parents, their bosses, their husbands, their upbringings, and their lack of money or education for why they don't have the lives they want. I started to realize that this mentality was the result of a rupture left unfelt. Rupture turns into depression and anger when it is not expressed, not moved through the body. It deadens a woman from the inside out.

I was raised in a world where women were dead to their own power. I watched every week for 18 years as Wilma sat angrily at the kitchen table for hours every Friday night, her coat buttoned up, waiting to be handed her wages by my father, who was working late and never thought about her schedule, her life, her time. I witnessed my mother never asking my father for what she wanted, but complaining bitterly and hating him quietly when he did things his way, rather than hers. I have heard thousands of women say things like, "There are no good men out there and that's why I am single," or "I have to stay at this job that I hate because I can't ever find another."

When a woman doesn't embody her rupture and move it through, she has turned away from the gift of life. Her lights are off, and her radiance goes dark.

THE 4 D's

It is not easy to choose radiance, especially in the midst of rupture. We do not yet have many models of women choosing this path. What we see instead are too many women who stumble blindly into what I call the 4 D's:

- Disenfranchisement (*I still don't get it or fit in; I'm an outcast*)

- Disapproval (*I disapprove of myself, everyone, and everything*)

- Devastation (*I have suffered devastating loss and can't get over it*)

- Depression (*I am so despondent and dejected I just can't engage*)

We learn to choose the 4 D's over radiance by watching generations of women before us. The conditioning toward disenfranchisement, disapproval, devastation, and depression is so insidious that we don't even experience it as a choice.

Over the years of teaching at the SWA, I have noticed that a woman can use almost any excuse to jump into the 4 D's. She might have a personal experience of shame or humiliation, such as divorce, or getting fired from a job, or not being able to find a partner. She might hear the good news of a friend having a baby—which she herself longs for—and suddenly judge herself for her own "flaws." The 4 D's often show up when a woman is the last of her group of girlfriends to get married or find partnership: she settles into depression or disapproval instead of finding herself right for walking a different path. Or if she can't find a job after college, she'll choose disenfranchisement instead of feeling hopeful or proud that she's holding out for work she loves.

When a woman has experienced rape or abuse of some kind, the humiliation is often so great she opts for devastation rather than confronting her attacker or reporting the crime. I once read an essay in *Harper's Bazaar* written by the singer Madonna. She wrote, "[New York] did not welcome me with open arms. The first year, I was held up at gunpoint. Raped on the roof of a building I was dragged up to with a knife in my back." She says she did not report the incident, because "You've already been violated. It's just not worth it. It's too much humiliation."

And that's *Madonna.* The definition of a powerful woman.

Why will 97 percent of all rapists never be incarcerated? Because too often we women slip into the 4 D's instead of taking action. We berate and disapprove of ourselves, taking the blame on behalf of our attacker. *I shouldn't have worn this short skirt. I shouldn't have flirted with those guys. I shouldn't have had anything to drink. I shouldn't have gone out. I deserved this. It was all my fault.* This devastating event leads to so much disapproval and shame that she becomes disenfranchised from herself and her world. The result is that her power is derailed, and she becomes hopeless.

The way back is very simple: she must cannonball herself into the heart of her rupture.

Then, she must choose to value and honor her radiance from inside the pain.

Radiance, in the midst of rupture. Radiance, even when there is no candle in the darkness, no light at the end of the tunnel. Radiance, as if her life depended on it. Rupture can never have its transformative way with her if she doesn't turn her radiance back on. The alchemy of the two, together, is what remakes her into a living legend.

REWRITING THE FAIRY TALE

What I see now is that I needed to be broken open. If not, I would have continued to live a small, girlish life, waiting for my prince to come rescue me. My whole life I had longed to be rescued. Since I was a tiny girl, being beaten by my brother, I had longed for a man to love me so much he would take all of my pain and suffering away. A man who would finally, finally take care of me.

Having that dream come true—and then losing it—threw me into a bottomless anguish. This anguish had been living inside of me since my childhood, but I hadn't been able to afford to feel it until now. Yes, I was grieving the loss of Tiitus. But I was also grieving the anguish of a two-, three-, four-, and five-year-old girl who no one stood up for. A girl who had not been saved from violence. Who had never been rescued.

Oh yes, this was a full-scale, custom-designed rupture, created especially for me by the Great Pussy in the Sky. Carefully orchestrated over the course of years. Over my whole life, really.

Rupture allows the part of a woman that she has outgrown to die and fall away. It updates the parts of us that feel helpless; like we need someone to do it for us. It forces us to take a seat firmly inside of our power. It is required for us to grow.

Rupture was required for me to make the School of Womanly Arts into the successful, high-functioning company it is today. I had no idea that I was capable of doing it on my own. If Tiitus had lived, I might *never* have done it. If he had lived, I would have wanted to quit my full-time job at the helm of the School and travel with him as he spoke at economic conferences around the globe. He wanted to take me to Berlin, to Finland, to Art Basel. I loved taking care of him and making sure he had whatever he needed. I had been interviewing chefs for him in the days before Niklas's accident—imagining the next season of our lives, filled with dinner parties, travel, and entertaining with delicious, healthy meals. If Tiitus had lived, I would never have had to create myself into the successful businesswoman and the creative force I've become. Necessity was the mother of my reinvention.

My life with Tiitus had to blow up, so *I* could blow up.

And in the process, I learned that reinvention and re-creation are a woman's birthright. We all go through cycles of up and down, continuing to create and re-create new iterations of ourselves as we grow and change through different life cycles and life experiences. Like Amaterasu and Demeter, we can all lose our way in the endless ruptures that life delivers. When Amaterasu was abused by her brother and shut herself in her cave, she was deep inside her devastation. It took the sisterhood of Ama-no-Uzume to "pussy" Amaterasu right out of that anguish with her naked dance of life. The dance allowed Amaterasu to move her emotions through her body. Only then could she recognize that as a woman she was the source of life and rebirth. Similarly, Demeter had lost herself to rupture when she lost her daughter. Baubo reminded her of her pussy power, which allowed her to not just step back into herself and restore life on earth, but to facilitate the rescue of her daughter from Hades.

Notice how, in these stories, the goddesses were rescued from their agony not by sympathy, empathy, or compassion, but by the pure unadulterated force of turn-on. It was their own devastation—and the radiance that broke open on the other side—that powered them back to sanity.

After I had crashed so completely, I had to remake a huge aspect of the School of Womanly Arts curriculum. Prior to Tiitus's death, I had no idea how to hold space for, or to navigate, the devastating losses that women experience. I had downplayed the importance, the *necessity*, of dropping into the depths of despair.

I took a lot of criticism from long-standing students for changing the curriculum to honor a woman's darkness as well as her light. But the changes I made mean that the SWA curriculum now fits perfectly with what a woman's soul wants and needs.

EMBODYING OUR EMOTIONS

Tiitus was never meant to be my happily ever after. He was meant to be the straw that broke the camel's back. His gift to me was not just the love we had, but also the *loss* of that love. The loss that led me to falling apart in a way I had never been able to do.

In designing and building the school—and an ongoing community for the women who pass through it—I had finally created a container that could hold me as all the pain of my childhood rose up and claimed me. A container that did not think my overwhelming, exploding, unstoppable grief was crazy. Our patriarchal culture does not honor grief. (Or rage. Or longing. Or jealousy. Or frustration—just to name a few.) We are all supposed to have plain vanilla emotions like happiness, compliance, and supportiveness. We're supposed to hold the big stuff at bay so we can punch our time cards and be productive and go to work and *get it done*.

After my experience with Tiitus, I learned that grief is sacred. It has an inherent intelligence and a time line that is perfect—whether it lasts a day or a year. My grief was not my enemy. It was my teacher. It had initiated me.

Prior to Tiitus, I had been holding my shit together. I was so well-defended that I couldn't even feel the feelings that were mine to feel. I pushed them away. I was still an uninitiated girl on the inside, and an uninitiated girl feels feelings very differently than an initiated woman. When a girl's heart is broken, she has no recourse and no resources. She seeks out the soothing arms of another to comfort her. When an initiated woman ruptures, she knows that the answer to her despair and desperation can be found in her own body. She may be in total devastation, but she knows how to steal her radiance back from the jaws of death. No one and nothing can take that away from her.

It was becoming clear to me that rupture was an important part of a woman's journey. Maybe *the* most important part. When winter descends and the leaves fall from the trees, they decay into mulch. That mulch fertilizes the soil of the next spring. Women are cyclical beings as well. We are designed to rupture in order to continually shed the skin that no longer fits us. Our pussies are designed to go through the entire cycle of rupture—through creation, shedding, bleeding, and preparation for re-creation—every single month. Through rupture we evolve into new iterations of ourselves. The tears of our devastation fertilize the soil of our evolution.

Mostly we have been taught that rupture victimizes us. But that's only because we don't know how to move our feelings through and find the radiance on the other side. Being turned on is a spiritual state. It is the golden thread that connects a woman to the meaning of her life, and to her desire. The consequence of turn-on is that a woman is plugged into her power source, connected to her divinity. Rupture, when turned off, is devastation and despair. Like Demeter, wallowing in the grief of the loss of her daughter, before she encountered Baubo. But turned-on rupture gives meaning to a woman's life. When Baubo flashed her pussy, it brought Demeter to her senses, and she turned back on. It's not that she stopped grieving; it's that she used the energy of her rupture to save her daughter and the world. In this way, rupture becomes the key to our evolution. It goes from being the perpetrator of our suffering to an honorable and necessary part of our sacred journey.

Learning to Swamp

And so, in the classroom, I began to research what it takes to reeducate a woman in the art of rupture. What I discovered is that, in order for a woman to experience rupture's gifts, she must learn to embody her pain fully, while being witnessed by other women.

Whether we've been raped or abused, have been divorced or lost a loved one, our ruptures have to be grieved *physically*, or they stay stuck inside our bodies. A woman can find her embodiment of rupture by listening to music that touches her soul and allowing her body to move as it wants to. I did this through my S Factor classes after Tiitus died. I learned to move my hips, my breasts, my ass, and to allow my deepest feelings to course through my being.

At the School of Womanly Arts we have a word for the process of moving emotions through our body: we call it Swamping.

I created this exercise for myself many years ago. At the time I was completing my sensuality training, and life was looking up. Yet I noticed I would still have periods when I felt down, and even hated myself. Periods when I felt completely at the mercy of my disapproval and depression.

In my sensuality training I learned the idea of "perfection": that every person is perfect exactly as they are. This concept dovetailed nicely with the research I had been doing on indigenous cultures, where I learned that spirit and matter are one. I was starting to see that truth all around me: it was impossible for me to not feel the presence of divinity when I saw a sunset, or held a gorgeous rose in my hand. I began to wonder if there could be divinity in the dark emotions I was feeling too. I wanted to experiment.

I decided that instead of hiding my emotions inside—which is what I had done my whole life—I would instead wear them on the outside. Truth was, I felt like garbage. So I went into the kitchen and pulled out a black trash bag. I pushed my head through the top and punched my arms through the sides until I was wearing it like a dress. I tied a babushka on my head and went to the fireplace and wiped some ash on my face. I blasted loud music, stomped around, and pounded pillows.

As soon as I did this, everything about my internal chemistry changed. I began to feel delighted with myself instead of hating myself. Having my outsides match my insides felt celestial. It gave me a whoosh of energy. It was also hysterically funny. And yes, I felt divine. When my roommates began to trickle home, they were all very entertained. And so was I! I was proud of myself, rather than ashamed.

I ended up gathering a whole line of "Swamp" clothing, including a "Psycho Bitch from Hell" T-shirt, camo pants, and biker boots. I began to notice that the more I greeted my inner bitch with warmth, love, and honor, the less frequently she visited. All she ever wanted was to be heard, and to be given her proper seat at the banquet table.

Swamping has not only stayed a regular part of my life, it's one of the core pieces of curriculum of the School of Womanly Arts. It's an excellent daily practice, because we all move through so many emotions inside of a single day. We are not all that different from toddlers, who collapse in frustration one moment, hurling themselves to the ground, only to pop up and go play on the swings with their friends the next moment. Toddlers have not been taught to stop embodying their emotions, so they do it naturally. But by the time they reach school age, most kids are thoroughly cut off from embodying the way they feel. By then they have been taught that their emotions are bad and wrong, and they begin to push them away.

Feeling our feelings is not considered an important value, because *nothing* of the feminine is considered important by the PWC. We have so deeply absorbed the bigotry and prejudice of the culture that we, too, have decided that feelings are messy, inappropriate, and unimportant. So when a woman has a big emotion, she finds herself wrong for it. But the feminine was *designed* as a deep feeler. In truth, huge emotions are fantastic—just like huge rainstorms are fantastic. Intense feelings cause us to grow, just like rain causes the earth to bloom.

Being shut down from our grief and rage deprives us of living our emotional and creative power. The practice of Swamping gives us that power back. We admit and embody the rupture. We roll around on the floor, rend our garments, throw our bodies into it. We experience and savor the full range of our feelings. If we want to live healthy lives as women, we need the space to grieve our asses off as often as we feel moved. Swamping gives us that opportunity.

Swamping is even more powerful when we do it in the presence of other women. This flows along with the rules of cliteracy: a woman requires attention in order to thrive. There is a part of her that will never unfold in a vacuum. The witnessing must be replete with approval and appreciation; no criticism, no disapproval, no judgment. Such witnessing cannot be done by just anybody. She must be witnessed by another woman. A woman who is a cheerleader, rather than a "fixer." A woman who will midwife her rupture.

My advanced students have been initiated as witnesses in this way. They know that every aspect of life is a gift, if it is regarded as such. That in order to live a life designed by our desire—which is a life of greatest service to the world—we must plug into the radiance of whatever is happening. The witness serves the same role as a doula at the birth of a baby. She is there to be the woman who knows; the woman who holds complete trust that her friend is in an important process of transformation. Who recognizes that the process must not be ameliorated, but rather encouraged. She knows the outcome will be spectacular, and she holds space for that result.

When we push our edges and fully express the storm that is passing through our being, we experience ecstasy and joy. Such an emotional storm clears out the cobwebs. Everyone who witnesses us—and Swamps *with* us—has the opportunity to clear out their own cobwebs too. The experience of moving powerful emotions through our bodies can take us to a place of power and beauty that we otherwise do not get to feel. It's the feeling of rapture, and it's just like the exquisite way the air feels after a generous rain.

Homework: Swamping

When we learn how to Swamp, we learn to ride the vicissitudes of life. Rather than feeling bad about feeling bad, we know what to do. Swamping comes in handy when we experience PMS; when we're overly tired or excited; and when we're stressed, scared, jealous, angry, heartbroken, or feeling any of the other dark emotions. We plug into our emotional truth, and then we embody the shit out of it. We dance. We scream. We bang on pillows, roll around on the floor, and wrestle with a girlfriend. In short, we let it move through us however it wants to.

This exercise will walk you through the steps to a Swamp. You'll need a journal, a big black trash bag, a pair of scissors, some loud music, some pillows and other props, and—if you really want to do it right—some witnesses to Swamp along with you.

Step 1: Before you start to Swamp, it's helpful to write out all the things that have upset you. (Note: For some women, the embodiment process is enough. But for others, writing down our feelings helps set the stage. Try it both ways and see which works best for you.)

Step 2: Get a trash bag. I'm serious—get a big, black trash bag. Cut a neck hole and arm holes, and pop it on like a dress.

Step 3: Put on some loud music. Don't have a favorite trigger song? May I recommend: Kelly Clarkson's "Addicted," if you are in a state of heartbreak; Rage Against the Machine's "Killing in the Name," if you are pissed at the world; or Kate Bush's "This Woman's Work," if you are sad and overwhelmed.

Step 4: Now take inspiration from a toddler you've known and embody your loudest emotion, as fully as you can. To get the rage going, try beating pillows or whacking a dishtowel against a wall. Try rolling around on the floor in frustration or sadness. Or lean your back against a wall and push your hips out, using the wall to wrestle with. Move your body the way your body wants to move.

Don't be afraid to feel or look awkward; it's part of the process. We don't have much experience embodying our emotions. You will get better at Swamping each time you do it. You'll be relearning something the little girl inside of you knows how to do but hasn't let herself. You'll be relearning how to really, truly feel your feelings. Just like a little kid having a tantrum or a meltdown doesn't last forever, there is a beginning, middle, and end to a Swamp. I recommend Swamping to music, as it creates a tight container to support your emotional experience. You can choose one, two, or three songs, depending how long you want your Swamp to be. Finish with a sensual song, as it ties a nice bow on the end of your emotional release and brings you back to turn-on.

Step 5: Consider being witnessed in your Swamp. I have a group of girlfriends who Swamp together once a month. We rent an empty dance studio, bring pillows and dishtowels, and create a great playlist. We each take turns yelling our Swamps into a microphone—saying out loud the things that upset us—and we cheer for one another's Swamps. We move and dance and crawl and stomp and beat the pillows and whip the walls with dishtowels. It is deeply fulfilling to roll around in the mud with others. We finish up by saying how we are the genius courtesans of all time, and then, finally, we share our desires. We are in and out in an hour, refreshed and renewed and ready to create anew.

Permission to Rupture

Feeling deeply is critical both for a woman's personal evolution and for the evolution of the world. Keeping a disapproving lid on our rich emotional lives results in debilitating depression and a sense of being disconnected from life, which results in all of the tragedy and abuse of our planet that we see all around us. But perhaps even more painfully, it results in women living in a near-constant state of numbness, unable to feel, much less reveal, the truth of our darkness.

When the feminine in a culture is repressed, the consequences are tragic. We end up with violence in schools, mass shootings, a mercenary corporate culture, and an environment on the brink of collapse. The game becomes power and profit, rather than humanity. We are passing the responsibility for feeling our pain down to our children and grandchildren, who will have to live with the consequences of our unwillingness to do so.

In his incredible book *The Smell of Rain on Dust*, Martín Prechtel observes that the reason our culture is so violent is that we do not know how to grieve. If we don't know how to embody our pain, we can't move on. And when we can't move on, the pain stays stuck inside us, creating all kinds of physical and emotional consequences.

The pain I experienced as a child haunted me my whole life. My posture was affected. I scrunched my shoulders up, as if I were going to be struck at any time. I was afraid of the dark, afraid of being stabbed or mugged. I had nightmares of being attacked. It took me years to move all of this pain out of my being, because it had been embedded there for so long.

Today I dance my emotions through my body, nearly every day. I dance at home by myself; I Swamp regularly with friends; I go to an S Factor class at least once a week. By feeling my feelings and moving them through my body every day, I stay in touch with my ever-changing emotions and ready to express whatever comes up. Regular Swamping does not spare a woman from rupture. But through it, she begins to understand that embodied rupture is an important part of her creative unfolding as a woman. So rather than shy away from rupture, she greets it open-armed. She knows rupture is as important to her rapture as winter is to spring.

My goal is to give *you* permission to rupture too—daily, if need be. To feel your deep emotions, and to embody them completely. This is not easy, because we have been taught to hide our deepest shame and our deepest darkness from both ourselves and each other. We've been taught not to be transparent, for fear of being shamed. But when a woman really learns to rupture well, she becomes connected with her deepest power. Ultimately, we learn to run in the direction of rupture as if it were Christmas morning. We know there is power to be excavated there.

Looking back, I am so grateful for every twist and turn of my story line. I now know the depth and breadth of the way I love, the way I grieve, the way I rise. And I have been able to restore thousands and thousands of women to loving themselves and their own stories—such that they are willing to experience every drop of their own emotional truth. What I've learned in this process is that rupture is the portal into the woman you're meant to be. No matter how huge or devastating your Swamp is, unimaginable beauty, power, and glory is always on the other side. For on the other side of Swamping—on the other side of rupture—is where we find our radiance.

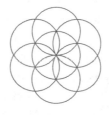

CHAPTER 7

RADIANCE

I pray for the courage
To walk naked
At any age
To wear red and purple,
To be unladylike,
Inappropriate,
Scandalous and incorrect
To the very end.

— GLORIA STEINEM

After the Tiitus rupture, I was cast out of the Garden of Eden. The only reason it did not kill me was that I already had a powerful connection to my turn-on and my radiance. It was my turn-on that allowed me to move decades of coagulated, unexpressed grief through my body. Being connected to my turn-on made living poetry of my grief, which actually fueled me. It allowed the woman I was becoming to take root inside of me.

But I cannot emphasize this enough: My pilot light had already been lit. I was already engaged with my pussy as a way of life. This meant that in making it through this rupture, as painful as it was, I always knew it was happening to serve me.

How I lit that pilot light is something I've hinted at throughout this book. It's a story that many of my students find confronting at first. (*I* found it confronting at first, myself).

In order to light my pilot light, I had to go on *a sensual journey*. And you—yes, you—will have to do the same.

Every woman's journey is different, but the common denominator is that the journey is about pussy, and it's about pleasure. Mine happened to be about female orgasm—learning to come better. But yours might be about something else. It could be dating men after years of being gay. It could be taking a female lover after years of being straight. It might include tantra classes, Orgasmic Meditation classes, or learning about BDSM. It might be taking a series of lovers after a divorce, taking S Factor pole-dancing classes, or studying sensuality by yourself or with a partner. It might simply be that you do all the exercises in this book.

Whatever you choose, the requirement is *to expand your sensual vocabulary beyond what you have known*. You must learn how to really, truly feel turned-on pleasure.

What do I mean by "turned-on pleasure"? I mean *pleasure whose source is pussy*. Take flirting, for example. Flirting causes turned-on pleasure, because when a woman flirts her pussy turns on. Her pussy turns on when she slowly swirls her tongue around a strawberry ice-cream cone. Or when she dances with her hips and ass. (As opposed to line dancing or river dancing, which mostly move her feet.)

The more a woman learns about her actual pussy, the more willing she is to play with her turned-on pleasure. The less she knows about her pussy, the more limited the range of her pleasure. Once she has learned to know and own herself sensually, she naturally embodies her turn-on and exudes radiance. She is more connected to her own divinity and her own inner GPS. Owning our pussy gives us room and permission to expand and explore other pleasures. Our pilot light is on, our spirit is engaged, so we can get off on an extraordinary piece of music, a fantastic meal, a gentle breeze, or a sunset. We have raised the bar for ourselves. We can hit heights of pleasure from, say, a sandwich at Katz's Deli—like that scene in *When Harry Met Sally*. (Only we *won't* be faking it.) We will know how to turn on our full-throttle experience of pleasure, whenever we like. That is the power, and the necessity, of getting a sensual education.

Here is the full story of mine.

My Sensual Journey

By the time I withdrew into my cave after college, I had very little interest in my pussy, and very little interest in orgasm. "Coming," as I would eventually refer to it fondly, was not something that took up much of my time or attention. And pleasure was something I had crossed off my to-do list many years before.

Don't get me wrong—I was always happy to have an orgasm. When my first boyfriend taught me what was possible, I was overjoyed. Whenever I went through periods of celibacy, I would test-drive my equipment once a month or so. You know, just to make sure it was working.

But I never really *thought about* orgasms. And I thought pleasure was unimportant, maybe even selfish. It never occurred to me that not only was it critical, it had a *profound* impact on who I was as a young woman. I thought of orgasm as something kind of nice, and kind of shameful. I was not a particularly promiscuous person, nor did I consider myself a particularly sexual person, so there were long expanses of time when I honestly forgot what was possible in my own body. Pleasure was eliminable. I mean, I had serious work to do!

What I *did* think about was confidence. Finding my purpose. Living my dreams. I desperately wanted to connect with my passion.

The search for my purpose is what took me into that acting class, where the teacher suggested I take a course in sensuality at More University. That class led to more classes, and eventually led to me moving in with the crazy, wonderful people who had become my teachers. They lived in something called a Morehouse:

a communal living space where sensuality was taught and practiced 24/7. It was called a Morehouse because, the philosophy went, if the world is good then more can only mean better. About 15 of us shared three floors of a brownstone, and we taught classes much like the sensuality course I had just taken.

The next step in my journey was to travel to California and take a class that was being given by the founder of More University, Dr. Victor Baranco. One section of this course was to watch my first DEMO—which you may recall stands for a Demonstration of Extended Massive Orgasm. I watched a man stroking his partner's clitoris for a few minutes, left the classroom, and promptly threw up. I was aware enough to realize that there must be something very powerful going on for me to have had such a dramatic response. When I returned to the room, everyone in the class had made a large circle, with one person on each side of the woman doing the demo. Each of those people was touching her leg, and the rest of the room was holding hands forming a circuit. I was encouraged to join the circle of hands, and as soon as I did I felt a bolt of energy run through my body. This disturbed me more than it delighted me. I really wanted nothing to do with this public display of orgasm.

But over the next few months I got more and more curious about the practice of extended orgasm. The technique had been developed by Dr. Baranco before he founded More University. He had been married to a woman named Susie, who had been inorgasmic. They went to all kinds of doctors to address the issue, with no luck. Victor was determined to solve this puzzle, and he experimented with a technique of manual genital stimulation. Instead of the typical sex act—which is generally all about the man getting off—he focused all his attention on his wife and simply stroked her pussy. He did it until he learned what she liked, how she responded, and which parts of her clitoris were the most sensitive. After years of research with Susie—and, later, with other couples—he realized that most people equated "sex" with "intercourse." And that intercourse was not an experience that favored a woman's pleasure.

Women, as we know today, are primarily orgasmic through clitoral stimulation—a fact that neither men nor women understood then and that resulted in very unhappy sex lives. He discovered that the clitoris was exquisitely sensitive and receptive. It had areas that were even more sensitive than others, like the upper left quadrant. A man simply had to learn to be attentive—and somewhat dexterous with his fingers—to deliver ecstasy to a woman's body. Which is actually not so simple, if he has never paid attention to what women want. So Victor began to teach classes in the practice and philosophy of pleasure. He also started a communal living situation where the object was to research communication, sensuality, and relationships. This was in the 1960s, and his movement grew rapidly. By the time I found the school, it had been in existence for about 30 years.

I had the opportunity to experience Victor's stroking technique with some of the men who lived at the New York Morehouse. Many of them had taken courses to learn how to deliver an extended massive orgasm to the body of a woman. I decided to try it. Understand, at this point in my life I had been sexually shut down for many years. Here I was, having my pussy stroked for 15 to 20 minutes at a time, with no obligation for any reciprocity. It was considered a totally gratifying experience for the stroker to put his attention on the woman he was stroking. An honor, actually. And the whole purpose of the session was to give her pleasure—there was no end goal of climax. It was pleasure for the sake of pleasure.

And it was a revelation, at least for me.

Turn-On Is a Choice

Finding my way to feeling my own pleasure was the first step toward true womanhood. It led me to have even greater confidence about my voice in the world. After many months of stroking sessions with my friends at More University, I felt powerful and important and valuable—feelings I'd never felt in my adult life.

Prior to my sensual journey, my doubts had been much louder than my talents. Now I was ready to step into my voice, my vision, and my desires in a new way. I spent two months on the main More campus in Lafayette, California, learning how to have an extended massive orgasm. When I got back, I became the orgasm evangelist in my house. I wanted as many stroking sessions as I could get in a day. I couldn't believe how good I felt, and how much energy and passion I had. I took more and more responsibility for running the different programs we were teaching, and we became more and more successful.

One of the most important lessons I was learning was that pleasure was a choice. Through many, many orgasmic sessions, I discovered that with the power of my intention I could enjoy any kind of stroke that a man gave me. Even outside of my stroking sessions, I was encouraged by the teachers to practice "turning on regardless of circumstance." Once I was assisting at a class called Advanced Sensuality, a six-week class covering communication skills and the difference between sensuality and sexuality. The exercises were done in pairs, and as an assistant, I was asked to step in if someone needed a partner. The final exercise of the six-week course was a kissing exercise. We taught three kinds of kisses—perfunctory, exploratory, and penetrative—and the students were to practice all three using a barrier of plastic wrap. There was a single man in the class named Will who was about 40 years old and overweight, with terrible grooming habits, eczema, and bad breath. Not surprisingly, he did not have a partner for the kissing exercise. The teacher of the course whispered to me that I was going to partner with him, as none of the participants was willing.

At first, I flat-out refused. I was revolted at the thought of kissing this man, even with the protective layer of plastic wrap. The teacher got angry. He said it was not just unfair but also unprofessional that someone who wanted to teach this material would have prejudices like that. He told me that my ability to turn on was powerful enough to trump my ego. It was my responsibility to make kissing Will the hottest kissing session of my life.

I was shocked by his suggestion, but the gauntlet had been thrown. I was not one to walk away from such a challenge.

It was a remarkable experience to simply *intend* to turn myself on. I had never made that choice before. And I found that once I turned on my *turn-on*, I turned on my divinity as well. I jumped into Will's lap, carefully secured the plastic in place, and started to kiss his pockmarked cheeks. It felt sweet and tender. Then I cranked my radiance up higher and began to kiss his lips—softly at first, then more deeply—eventually touching my tongue to his. Even with the plastic barrier, I found myself seriously turned on. Through my turn-on, Will became a child of God in my eyes. I could suddenly see and feel the beauty of him.

The experience became sacred to me. I'd had no idea that getting turned on was a choice—*a choice I could make anytime I wanted to*. My ability to get turned on that day was not about Will. Turn-on was not about *any* man. It was about *me*. It was about my connection to my spirit, my radiance. I felt free and powerful and confident in a way I had never known before. I felt divine.

Turn-on was something I had been taught to keep under wraps, as if standing in my radiant life force meant I would be diminished or disadvantaged. That stance turned off my interior light. Not only for me, but for the world I inhabited.

In some way, every woman is living the stories of Amaterasu and Demeter. Each of us has had some kind of rupture—be it incest, rape, verbal abuse, being ignored, what have you. What happens as a consequence is that we women get *angry*, and we turn off our radiance. We go wandering the earth, unwilling to light the world up with our life-giving turn-on. We—and the entire world—suffer the consequences. We do the only thing we know how to do: we make the unconscious choice to cut ourselves off from our own radiance. Repressed radiance turns into anger. Because we don't have an external outlet where we can express it, we turn that anger toward ourselves—where it settles in as depression and sadness.

Want to know something that makes a woman *really* angry? When this choice is pointed out to her. When she's invited to release the anger and reclaim her radiance instead. She gets furious at the thought of reigniting the gift of her turn-on, because she has taken sides against it. She was hurt so young and had to turn herself off to stay protected. Now she is infuriated at the very thought of a different choice.

It brings to mind the first generations of Chinese women who were told they could not bind their feet. Binding the feet of upper-class women had been a practice for centuries, as tiny feet were viewed as attractive to men. The custom meant that women were utterly dependent; they could barely walk after their feet were bound. It took centuries of protests and finally a government edict to keep women from binding their daughters' feet. Women *wanted* to cripple themselves for the sake of being attractive to men. Self-defilement on behalf of men continues to this day, as the statistics for female genital mutilation attest. Somewhere in the world, women are mutilating their young daughters' pussies *right this very minute*. Women initiate and carry out the cutting, and it is considered a source of honor.

We long for the thing that feels culturally and historically comfortable, even when that thing is self-defilement and self-abuse.

In a powerful essay called "Uses of the Erotic: The Erotic as Power," feminist writer Audre Lorde writes about a force that she calls the "erotic"—which is the same thing I call "radiance" or "turn-on." She says:

> As women, we have come to distrust that power which rises from our deepest and non-rational knowledge. We have been warned against it all our lives by the male world, which values this depth of feeling enough to keep women around in order to exercise it in the service of men, but which fears this same depth too much to examine the possibilities of it within themselves. So women are maintained at a distant/inferior position to be psychically milked, much the same way ants maintain colonies of aphids to provide a life-giving substance for their masters.

Word, Audre.

What she does not include in this essay is the fact that cutting off from our radiance is an *inside job*. We women are the ones who cut ourselves off, and it is only in the company of women that we can reclaim what was once ours. The courtesans were women who were not fueled by their circumstances, because their early circumstances were usually dire. They were fueled by their turn-on, which made them radiant. This is what happens when I gather women for my SWA classes. This reclamation ricochets into every corner of a woman's life, restoring her sense of being in control of her destiny, easefully overcoming life's obstacles, and carrying a sense of spirited radiance into all her endeavors.

The tricky and elusive problem we face is that because there is no encouragement of radiance in this culture, and no modeling from one woman to another, it is incredibly difficult to presence the importance of connecting to our inner power source. We will find billions of way more important things to do.

When in truth, there is nothing more important than feeling radiant.

Nothing.

Sounds crazy, I know. But when we feel radiant, we get everything we have always wanted. We feel powerful, confident, and in control. Like the courtesans in whose lineage we are walking, we know who we are in time and space. We know we are not victims, but the heroines of our own lives. The stars of our show. Walking hand in hand with our divinity, guided by the GPS.

When we are not standing in our radiance, on the other hand, we are like lamps that are not plugged in. Utterly useless to ourselves and others. We function as creatures of service and caretaking, rather than living, breathing reflections of the divine.

Which explains why so many women wind up in cleanup and caretaker roles in this world. Why so many women settle for pay that is not commensurate with our talents, training, or interest. When we are not connected to our innate life force, we are directionless. We use other people's expectations in place of our own internal compass. When we are not plugged into our divinity, we feel inadequate—and therefore we're willing to accept inadequacy.

Sister, we do not have time to live as less than who we are. We do not have time to allow the PWC to keep the blinders on our eyes. The world requires the voice of radiant, awakened women who are turned on. Our voices are needed to re-create our futures and the futures of our sons and daughters. It's time for you to reconnect. It's time to prioritize your radiance.

It's time for you to take a sensual journey of your own.

Your Sensual Journey

So how do we learn to access this radiance that is ours for the taking? *We must reclaim our sensuality.* And befriending your pussy is the way. You must put her at the controls, which means doing basically the exact opposite of everything you have been taught to do by the PWC. Your path does not have to look anything like mine, but you *must* forge a path of pussy reclamation for yourself. You must become cliterate through practice, attention, and discovery. You must plug into the spiritual and sensual circuitry that sources your radiance and connects you to your GPS.

The definition of a sensual journey is quite subjective, but there's a formula I've discovered over the years. First, there's a spark of turn-on. Turn-on is like a virus—it's contagious. Usually a woman catches this spark from another woman. One whose radiance is palpable, who has something she, herself, does not have. Her unexpectedly strong desire to experience that turn-on overrides her resistance; she can't help but follow it, even though the road looks dangerous. The road looks dangerous because it requires her to plug back in and engage with her very own pussy. As soon as she does, however, what looked dark and terrifying is revealed to be magical and infinitely pleasurable. She's reconnected her to her own sensuality. Plugged back into her power source, she begins to glow with a radiance that has always been inside of her. She has become the same type of woman who first sparked her curiosity, her turn-on, at the beginning of the journey. Her pilot light is on—finally—and it can't be extinguished again.

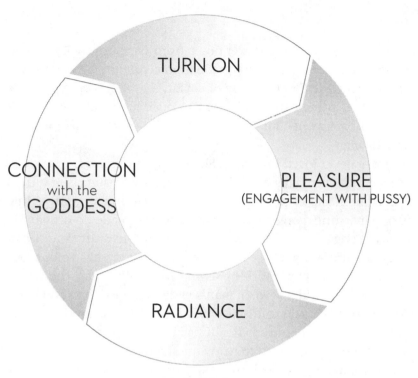

Cycle of Radiance

So how do we find that initial spark of turn-on to launch our very own sensual journey? I have wonderful news for you: You're already on your way! You picked up this book. Something sparked your curiosity, and picking up the book was your leap of faith. Moreover, you've made it through the first chapters of this book, all about *pussy*. In other words, the connection has been made.

The sensual journey is the equivalent of taking pussy out for a drive. See how she operates. Play with her gearshifts. It's only after you slip your key into your own ignition, turn that baby on, and take her for a spin that you can safely invite passengers to come on board.

I have shared my own sensual journey with you, but every woman's journey is unique. Here are two stories from students of mine, whose sensual journeys look very different from my own.

Joyce

Joyce is a 55-year-old composer from New York City. When she first came to the Mastery graduation ceremony as a guest, she was overwhelmed with a sense of *not* having what was so palpable among the women there. She was so overwhelmed she couldn't even talk to anyone. But she knew she wanted what these women were having.

Joyce never loved her pussy. She never even knew it was something that required her attention. After taking Mastery, she started a morning ritual of pulling out her handheld mirror and saying, "Good morning, gorgeous!" to her pussy. She made no other conscious changes. Yet somehow, things started to shift. She began dressing differently, allowing herself to show off her voluptuous hips and booty. One morning as she was walking on the Lower East Side, a Hasidic Jewish man—wide-brimmed hat and all—stopped in his tracks and said, *"HELL-OOO!"* This kind of thing had not been happening to her. It had been a long time since anyone noticed or responded to her when she walked down the street. But this man was turned on by her turn-on. Soon nearly every man she passed gave her his attention. It didn't feel lewd or offensive; it was lovely and made her feel powerful. She was turned on by her *own* turn-on! It brought her so much joy.

She found whenever she remembered to say good morning to her pussy, she would have an extraordinary day. She began finding time in her day for dance breaks and writing. She tried new, inventive, and daring things at work. But the biggest change she reported was that she stopped being in disapproval of herself. When Joyce is standing in her turn-on, she feels capable. She's confident her desires will be met—whether by herself, her students and colleagues, or by men.

Kimberly

A physician by trade, Kimberly began listening to her pussy only after a series of punishing circumstances. Her grueling years in medical school and residency had resulted in a complete pussy disconnect. She internalized limiting beliefs inherent in the PWC-driven medical community: "Playfulness and silliness will be your enemies to finding success in life." "Women should not be overtly sexual." "As a woman, you will be held to higher standards than men just to be accepted." "Having a strong sexual desire will keep you from being taken seriously." "Your actions will never have as much value as a man's." As a result of these messages, she took a deep dive into a dark corner of her existence, hiding her true self from the world.

Meanwhile, she was plagued for over a decade by severe endometriosis, a painful disorder associated with menstruation, and eventually had a complete hysterectomy. She'd become a physician in order to teach people about how their bodies worked, and how to increase pleasure in their physical health and sexuality. Instead, she was working on an inpatient unit at a hospital, spending her days fighting with insurance companies. Worse, most of the care she was administering was just patching over much deeper problems.

By the time she came to the School of Womanly Arts, Kimberly was physically and spiritually drained.

In beginning to explore her connection to her own pussy, practicing the Tools and Arts every day, and receiving the support of a sisterhood community, she was able to quit her job and do what she always wanted to do. She wrote a book on male sexual issues and started a blog. She also found that her connection to her pussy allowed her to look at and feel the depths of her anger, which is something she'd always repressed. She realized she did not have to be afraid of this power. She began to trust that her feelings were right and important. She used the Swamping exercise from the last chapter to process her anger, and she realized that feeling everything that was hers to feel led her to more happiness than she'd ever experienced. She was no longer willing to silence her pussy. In her words, "My pussy reclamation has been in finding her voice—the one I thought needed to be silenced, the one I thought no one wanted to hear, the one I feared no one would pay attention to. That same voice is the one that has the power to change lives. To me, this reclamation means being myself with no disclaimers or excuses. It means not needing permission to say what's important or to ask for guidelines around how to say it. My reclamation is becoming aware that my voice has power and meaning, and is the only way I will create my desired life for me, and those around me."

RADIANCE AS OUR BODY BIRTHRIGHT

There is a natural consequence for a woman when she takes the time and attention to learn herself sensually. She becomes an endless source of radiance, her whole life long. She has an internal glow that is timeless and undiminishable by age.

We have come to expect that tiny babies and little kids are radiant. They are radiant because they are relaxed in their self-love. They take enjoyment in themselves, their cute bodies, and the gift of being alive. Yet girls tend to lose their radiance over time, as they grow older. Why? Because we begin to absorb the judgments of the culture, almost all of which are negative toward women. Negative judgment kills radiance. If we think we aren't pretty enough or thin enough or smart enough, our inner light dims. Disapproval, doubt, and depression take their toll. The older we become, the more we learn to disconnect from our pussy intuition, and the more and more wrong we find ourselves.

We don't realize that it's our enjoyment of ourselves and our bodies that creates, and re-creates, radiance inside of us. The last place we are taught to look for our turn-on is our own bodies. Yet a woman who is turned on to herself and her life is a woman in her highest power.

We have all seen people, or been people, in the first blush of love. What radiance! Every cell of our being feels thrilled to be alive. We are sensually vibrant and pulsing. But the chemistry of falling in love is temporary. Is it possible to keep the glow of love radiating through us every day, our whole lives? Is it possible to fire up our own furnace, without needing someone else to do it for us? When women are in the company of other radiant women, turn-on is a constantly renewing resource. We fuel and replenish each other. We remind one another of the eternal truth that turn-on is required for a woman to live at optimum health and fitness.

When a woman is turned on, she is empowered with her own elemental rightness. Cliteracy rewires her to *expect* radiance as her natural resting state. When a woman gets turned on, she tunes in to her own magnificence, into her sense of deserving all that is wonderful in this life. She becomes radiant, the way a woman is supposed to be. An innately feminine wisdom begins to emerge, allowing her to trust herself, her voice, and her experience. This sense of trust eludes a woman who has never connected her body and soul in this way. It may be uncomfortable at first; Joyce, whose story you just read, was so confronted by the turn-on in the room at the Mastery graduation ceremony that she could barely speak. But in time, this turn-on is like a wildfire: it will catch fire in others' bodies too. I cannot emphasize this enough. *Each of us becomes a force for positive change and evolution in the world, simply by getting turned on.* A radiant woman is a woman in her highest power, a woman who is bringing what she is meant to bring to the world.

GOING HIGHER

I saw this modeled for me in an extraordinary way the day I did the demo for Vera Bodansky. As you may recall, while Steve and I taught the class and did the demo, Vera was undergoing medical tests. As soon as the course was finished we raced to the hospital, just as the doctors were coming into her room with the test results. They told us she had colon cancer, and possibly liver cancer.

Steve promptly fainted, our Cuban friend Carmen screamed out loud, and I froze. Vera remained calm. She turned to all of us with a radiant smile.

"Well, then," she said, "we will just use this as a chance to go higher."

To "go higher," in Vera's terminology, meant to take full advantage of the experience. It meant to stay in her radiant turn-on, which enabled her to see the cancer as a gift—and to use the opportunity to surrender even more fully to the experience of her life. She intended to find pleasure, meaning, and transformation in the process, and to take the rest of us along with her.

Vera was 65 years old and had been studying and teaching about orgasm for more than 30 years. When you have orgasm that deep in your body, you understand something about the truth of life. Vera knew that she could take *any* circumstance, good or bad, and use it as a vehicle for pleasure and transformation. She knew this because that's what orgasm had done for her, over and over. She had the confidence of a woman who knows her own regenerative, restorative power.

In the world of the feminine, encountering a rupture is not about survival; it's not about making lemons into lemonade. It's about using breakdown as our cue to take an even deeper sense of responsibility—to acknowledge that we, ourselves, are the creatrixes of our own stories. In other words, *we actually created the lemons*. We drew in the perfect circumstances to help ourselves unfold more lush and gorgeous layers of who we are as women. We created this situation to step more powerfully into the women we were born to become.

There is no such thing, in nature, as a rupture without redemption. Vera was living, breathing proof that there was the potential for perfection in every occurrence, no matter how dire it might seem. I found this breathtakingly beautiful, and I determined to become an even more vigilant student of this practice inside my own body and life.

Because Vera was ill, I took her place and co-taught all of the private sessions she had been teaching with Steve. I had the unexpected experience of teaching more than 100 sessions in the next three months. I saw women's bodies of every shape and size, and I was taken inside the heart of the sensual longings of so many diverse people. I learned how much pain and ignorance people have about sensuality, and how deeply wrong so many people feel about their sex lives. I also learned how proud and joyful men become when they are able to give their women pleasure. And I saw how radiant women become when they feel more pleasure than they could have ever imagined for themselves.

Vera recovered completely. She returned to California after she became strong enough to travel, and after a difficult round of chemo, she gradually resumed life as usual and was restored to her full health. She has been unflagging in her support of me and my work, and she encouraged me all along the way as I grew the School of Womanly Arts and wrote my first book.

And that is the genius of pussy. Female orgasm is a living, human model for experiencing the inherent divinity in all things. Through orgasmic practice I learned to enjoy each and every stroke my pussy received, with no goal in mind. Approaching my life in the same way is, from my perspective, the best way to live. Unless they live in the body, ideas like "the Goddess lives in all of us" and "everything is divine" are just intellectual theories. In this way pussy engagement is the pathway home, to where our divinity becomes an alive experience inside of us, ready to be transmitted to others.

Radiance comes from a woman knowing and owning the truth: that she is the portal to life. Just like the sun, her light is always on. There is somebody home. She is connected to the elemental life force. She knows herself to be the altar that connects this world to the world of the Goddess—the world of the divine. But just like any altar, the candles have to be lit for the holiness to be present. An altar without candles is just a shelf. A woman without radiance is devoid of her divinity.

The courtesans were radiant women; they turned on amid lives that were rife with rupture. But radiance comes in many different styles. Mother Teresa was a radiant being: she lived the love she had in the world. You can see her glow through photos, and in the way she seemed to have an endless source of energy for helping those in need. Actress Katharine Hepburn is another example of a woman who lived her radiance. She was openly known to be Spencer Tracy's mistress. This meant she had to powerfully and pridefully step into a role that women have long been humiliated for choosing. Radiant women often choose atypical, unusual, and controversial paths. They have broken the norms of the PWC and have chosen to follow their own pussy truth instead. In the process, they inspire the rest of us to live lives that are authentically ours—without disapproval, self-hatred, or shame.

Homework: The Holy Trinity

Finding and reclaiming our radiance is a choice we must make daily. After much research in my favorite lab—the SWA classroom—I have developed a technology for choosing radiance in a moment-by-moment way. Reaching for turn-on when our lives feel turned upside down is not the common choice, but that doesn't mean it has to be hard. Get familiar with doing a Holy Trinity on the daily, and you'll see what I mean.

This exercise requires a partner—ideally a friend, a Sister Goddess who is walking the same path of pussy reclamation. I will tell you more about SGs in the final chapter of this book. But for now, choose someone who feels like a safe recipient of your truth—someone you know will listen without judgment or criticism. This exercise only takes five minutes when done right, and it can be done over the phone or, in a pinch, via text or e-mail. Recommended dose: once or more per day, as needed.

Whether you're in the midst of an especially difficult day, sunk deep into the 4 D's, or feeling light as a feather, you will now prepare to brag about yourself, find something to be grateful for, and name something you want.

Step 1: Brags

The first stage of the Holy Trinity is to give three brags. A brag celebrates the goodness in your life. It's something you love, value, and are proud of—about yourself, your life, or your world. This is a practice of finding something *right* about yourself, which is quite the opposite of what the PWC has us women focused on most of the time. Pick three instances of success, glory, power, and radiance, and then brag them. For example:

I brag that I have a hot lover who traveled two hours just to be with me last night.

I brag that when my kid brought home a report card with two D's, I didn't freak out.

I brag that the meeting I ran at the office yesterday went easily, and I felt confident the whole time.

Step 2: Gratitudes

Now's the time to thank the Goddess for the blessings she's showering upon you. For even in the midst of a knock-down, drag-out rupture, the radiant woman knows how to appreciate her experience. Gratitudes come in all shapes and sizes, so just choose three that feel alive to you. For example:

I'm grateful that when my car got sideswiped last night, I wasn't inside of it.

I'm grateful that my boyfriend brought me dinner tonight so I didn't have to cook.

I'm grateful for the rain, which is bringing my garden back to life.

Step 3: Desires

The final stage of the Holy Trinity is to ask for three things you want. Desire is the way the Goddess speaks through us; you can think of naming your desires as taking dictation for the Divine. Don't buy into the PWC's idea that desire is selfish! Desire is the map a turned-on woman trusts most. Claiming what you want is not just a fun exercise, it's your responsibility as a radiant being. Be sure to get really specific—the more details you provide, the more likely the universe will know exactly how to answer! Here are a few desires to get you started:

I want to finish working on this report in time to go take an S Factor class tonight at six o'clock.

I want to have a summer house in Amagansett, no more than a five-minute drive from the beach, with at least four bedrooms so I can invite my best women friends for the weekend.

I want to take weekly guitar lessons and set aside at least 30 minutes to play and sing every day.

We women have no idea that radiance lives within us. That no matter what happens in our lives—no matter how horrendous, devastating, hurtful, or destructive—we are wired to take that rupture and *go higher*. It is not just our nature, it is our physiology.

When we are turned on, our clit knows how to keep going higher. She can take us up with light strokes, medium strokes, or heavy strokes—whatever comes her way. That's the nature of being a turned-on woman. When we do not know our physiology, and are not surrounded by women who know theirs, we can't connect with this innate truth that we are wired for continual creation and re-creation, no matter what. We never have to lose our sense of connection to our own power and divinity, because our radiance is innate. But we don't *know* it's innate, because we've been taught to fear and run away from the very source of our power: our pussy.

After the loss of Tiitus, which was the straw that broke this camel's back, I was in a state of rupture so profound I could not find my way out. The first thing I did was take up residence in the swamp, so I could really give myself a chance to grieve for all that I had lost. I grieved the loss of our love, the loss of our friendship. I grieved feeling helpless as a businesswoman. I grieved that no one was there to rescue me. I grieved being a single mom, wondering if my love and attention was enough to raise my daughter. I grieved my troubled past, and all the pain and hurt that I could never afford to feel. In the process I discovered something very unexpected. I found that within my embodied grief, there was radiance. I felt beautiful and pure in my devastation. I felt no rush to move from this space. It was mine: my love, my anguish, my loss, *mine*. I had lived; I had loved and been loved by an extraordinary man. The way I connected with my radiance again was to pour turn-on into the embodiment of that grief.

For example, a few weeks after Tiitus's death, I had a private client who was coming in for a session. I was having a very emotional day, and I didn't know how I was going to get through it. But instead of canceling, I put on a pair of thigh-high black boots, booty shorts, and a tank top. I turned on some music and I danced, moving the grief through me in a sensual way. I circled my hips and arched my back. I poured the sensual into my sadness. The result was a sense of powerful radiance. I had restored myself by plugging into my turn-on. I could feel ownership of my story again, rather than feeling like a victim of it. Emerging, I delivered an even more robust and passionate session for my client than I could have imagined. Turn-on had transformed my grief into a benediction.

The viewpoint I'm presenting here requires an extreme sense of responsibility for one's life. But the reward is an extreme sense of ownership of one's destiny. If we are the co-creatrixes of our lives, then we are never lost, never off the path, never alone.

Our cultural connection to the Divine Feminine is the radiant woman. A turned-on woman is a portal to the Goddess, for herself and others. We can actually *see and feel* radiance through her. She emanates it like light or heat, and the attraction is undeniable. All it takes is to approve of our own sensual fire and how much we enjoy the experience of being women. Which begins with that leap of faith: trusting our pussy. Once we know our own pleasure, we are turned on to and tuned in to our divinity. From that spot, radiance is not only possible, it's inevitable.

And there's no more central location for a woman's radiance to come to life than in relationship with those she loves. A turned-on woman has the ability to shine her light on everyone in her life, especially her chosen partner. In this next chapter, we are going to explore what radiant relationship means—and how to create one (or many!) in your life.

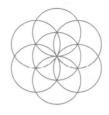

CHAPTER 8

RADIANT RELATIONSHIP

How is man to recognize his full self,
his full power, through the eyes of an incomplete
woman? . . . When woman is lost, so is man. The truth
is, woman is the window to a man's heart and a
man's heart is the gateway to his soul.

— JADA PINKETT-SMITH

We all long for love.

We all want to be seen and known and appreciated for every drop of everything we are. For some of us, the natural outcome of this longing is marriage or partnership. For others, alternate styles of intimacy are more gratifying or appropriate. Creating radiant relationship means choosing a relationship (or relationships) that will best serve your radiance. This definition might change and evolve over a lifetime. Luckily, we live in an age where there are many options open to us. We no longer have to create a relationship that conforms to other people's expectations; we can make our own choices, choices that serve our deepest desires and longings.

I was raised by parents who had a very traditional partnership. My mother kept the home and my father supported us. What I witnessed and experienced was not something I wanted to replicate. Traditional marriage felt stifling and limiting to me, and I was much more interested in freedom and space and exploration than I was in becoming a wife. Unlike my mother or grandmother, I grew up in a time when a woman *could* choose freedom and space. I was able to support myself, and my child, without the help of a partner. As a result, my requirements for relationship are born not out of economic necessity, but out of desire. I have more choice—which is both scary and wonderful. Scary, because I have no role models for the desires I've discovered to be mine. (They are nontraditional, to say the least.) And wonderful, because there are no limits on what I can experience or with whom.

Your desires may be strictly traditional, and perfect for you. Or they may be entirely unprecedented in your world. Once our radiance is turned on, it doesn't really matter anymore. We are always following where the GPS is pointing, trusting our pussy as we go.

But this means we must choose a relationship that serves our radiance first. Why? As they say, when the mama is happy, everyone's happy. Unfortunately, most women have no idea what makes them happy. We were brought up to pay attention to the happiness of our husbands, fathers, mothers, and children—but not our own. This is why so many relationships fail. The woman has gotten the message that to keep her relationship alive, she must devote all her time and energy in service to others. If she sacrifices herself for the good of her husband and kids today, she might someday be good enough to get hers.

In reality the opposite is true. By giving away everything she has, a woman loses access to her power source. And *she* is the power source of every relationship she is in. Just as we would all perish if the sun never rose again, a turned-off woman slowly destroys her relationships. *A relationship cannot be healthy when the woman is not turned-on, radiant, and happy.*

Guys are pretty simple. They're happy in their relationships if the women in their lives are happy with *them*. It's we women who are complicated. Complicated because we've forgotten the ancient truth that our pleasure is our power source. We were raised on a bunch of fairy tales that tell us if we slave away hard enough, eventually our fairy godmother will show up and dress us for the ball. Or that if we behave passively and look pretty enough, a prince is bound to come kiss our ruby lips and bring us back to life.

All of us grew up on our fair share of Cinderella, Sleeping Beauty, and Snow White. Women who were mostly in a coma, waiting and waiting and waiting for that prince to come. I know thousands and thousands and thousands of women who are still waiting like this to be rescued. Some of them are old enough to be the prince's grandmother by now. I want you to consider entertaining the idea that those fairy stories you were raised on might not be even a tiny dot true. Women are the center of everything, including our own happiness. And, in fact, men cannot really even help very much in the rescue department. They are busy trying to find their own way in the world, without the light of the feminine on the inner or the outer. We women need to reach inside and rescue ourselves, which is oh-so-possible with a community of sisterhood supporting us. Once we have community in place, building a relationship with a partner is so much easier. Our sisters fuel us as we fuel our relationships.

Radiant relationship requires us to unlearn basically everything we've ever known about relationship. It's about designing the way we relate so it serves our turn-on first—trusting that it's our turn-on that feeds the men in our lives, not the other way around. It's about taking full responsibility for our own happiness, even while we're with others. It's about learning what lights us up and turns us on, so we can use our radiance as a road map for creating wonderful relationships in our lives. All of which begins with the most important relationship any woman will ever have: the relationship with her very own pussy.

The Story of Biff

How is it that we women have been so poorly educated about what makes a relationship work? Let me weave you a tale to explain.

Once upon a time there was a sweet little girl. Her next-door neighbor was a sweet little boy around the same age. His name was Biff.

Like every girl in her neighborhood, she grew up running around, playing in the park, and enjoying her friends. She knew she had a nose and knees and eyes and ears—and *nothing* "down there." Like every boy in the neighborhood, Biff grew up running around, playing in the park, and enjoying his friends. He knew that he had a nose and knees and eyes and ears, and that he had a *penis* "down there."

The two grew up and went to nursery school together, and then kindergarten. Our girl still had nothing, and Biff still had a penis. But they were just little kids, so who cared what they had? Years passed, and they continued to play together after school. Sometimes basketball, sometimes dolls. Sometimes heading to the playground. Frequently running in and out of each other's houses for peanut butter sandwiches.

Years happily passed, and the little neighbors were now in middle school. One day, the girl walked outside and saw Biff waiting for her, as usual. But something about today was different. As they walked home, she turned to look at him. He had recently just shot up a few inches. He was coming from baseball practice, and she noticed for the first time that his arms rippled with new muscles. The sun caught the brightness of his big brown eyes; a lock of his hair fell over his forehead, and he flung it back just like a rock star. Suddenly and unexpectedly, the hair on her arms stood on end. She felt chills run up and down her spine. Their eyes met, and she stared at his beautiful face. How had she never noticed before? As his gaze locked with hers, he seemed caught in the same spell. As if enchanted, he reached down and placed a sweet and tender kiss on her lips. Then, with a quick, blushing "Bye!" he headed home.

She stood frozen at the end of her driveway. What had just happened? She was overcome by a feeling she'd never felt before. Her lips felt swollen and bee-stung. Her body was vibrating and her knees were weak. This was incredible, wonderful, phenomenal. It was . . . in a word . . . *everything.* She had never felt so alive. She could hear a movie soundtrack swelling in the background, foretelling her destiny. The prince had come! And his name was Biff. *Oh my God, this was the most wonderful thing in the entire world since the dawn of time!*

She immediately ran into her house, taking the stairs two at a time, locking herself in the bathroom to look at her freshly kissed lips. She wondered if anyone would notice. Did she look different? Could people tell that she was *a kissed woman?* She ran to her room, planning her outfit for the next day. She had to dress hot so Biff would notice her and kiss her again. (And then . . . who knows??) She could barely sleep all night. Even though he had never called her before, she kept waiting for the phone to ring, or for a text to come in. She needed some sign to tell her that this *major event* had really happened to her.

At school the next day, every time she even *thought* of passing him in the hall she felt a rush of anticipation. She could barely eat her lunch, she was so excited about their walk home from school. All during math class, she kept doodling *Mr. and Mrs. Biff* in the margins of her notebook, barely absorbing anything the teacher said.

Biff had baseball practice after school, so he was not heading home right away. She decided to go watch him practice. She kept trying to get his attention—waving at him and yelling, "Biff! Over here!!!" But he was too absorbed in his game to notice. Or was he ignoring her?

When practice was over, he left with the guys. She did not let that stop her. She trailed after them, calling out, "Biff! Wait up!" Even *she* knew she was kind of making a fool of herself, but she didn't care.

She cared about one thing, and one thing only.

To feel *that feeling* again.

That feeling of being so alive, so wanted, so lit up, so deeply *herself.*

That feeling she thought had come from Biff.

She had no idea that all of that aliveness, turn-on, power, and radiance came from *her*. What she'd actually experienced was her first taste of her own divine radiance—amplified, because someone was reflecting it back to her.

This is a point of deep confusion for all women. We've been taught our entire lives that a man makes us feel a certain way. That the man has all the power in a relationship. We're set up to believe that in relationships the man chooses the woman. Actually, it's the other way around. Look at the animal world. An old tomcat just sits around napping in the sun until a female cat in the neighborhood goes into heat. When he gets even the slightest whiff of her turn-on, he's clawing at the screen door to get in. She is the source of the desire, the erotic pull, the turn-on. It is her radiance that brings all the boys to the yard.

It works the same for men and women. Women set the course of desire. If she doesn't want it, it ain't happening. And if she does want it, he will eventually succumb. The turn-on comes from her, not him. It may feel mutual, but it's not going to happen unless she gives the green light. Yet because we women have believed it to be the other way around for so many thousands of years, it's really, really difficult for us to see another viewpoint. I mean, how do you teach the sun that she's the sun? Imagine it. She's looking around, and she sees light everywhere. She thinks, *I'm on the same ride as all of you! I'm not anything special.* She is the only one who can't see it, because she is it.

Back to our story. The only thing our little girl wanted was to feel that feeling again. And of course she thought if she just ran after Biff he would be the one to give her the feeling.

So she chased him relentlessly.

And he ran away relentlessly.

For her part, she did not realize that she had tossed all of her magnificent, divine power into the lap of a 14-year-old boy who couldn't even match his own socks. For his part, he couldn't understand what was happening to his best buddy from next door. It was just a little kiss, after all! She had been so *normal* the day before, and now she was acting just plain crazy.

Each of us is that little girl. We run hopelessly and helplessly after the boy (or girl) next door, believing someone else to be the source of our power, radiance, and pleasure. And if this particular Biff slips away? No problem. We move on to the next . . . and the next . . . and the next. There are so many Biffs in the world, we will never go through them all. Biff will not always be a boy—Biffs come in any and every age. Biff won't even always be a person. We use The Story of Biff as a metaphor and "to Biff" has become a verb. Sometimes we Biff a school we *really, really have to get into.* Or a job we *must* to have in order to feel right about ourselves. We might Biff a baby, or a marriage. A house on the right block, a certain type of car, or membership in a prestigious club.

We Biff anything outside of ourselves that seems like a source of power. If we believe, even on a subtle level, that we *need* that outside power source, we are Biffing. Why do we do this? Because we were *taught* to. The PWC has taught us not to believe in our innate pussy wisdom, our natural intelligence, our radiance. Our culture has taught us that we, as women, are powerless.

Feminism doesn't solve Biffing. Equal opportunity doesn't solve Biffing. Therapy doesn't solve Biffing. An Ivy League education doesn't solve Biffing.

There was a story in *The New York Times* a couple of years ago describing how the women at Harvard Business School are lagging far behind the men, both academically and socially: "Women at Harvard did fine on tests. But they lagged badly in class participation, a highly subjective measure that made up 50 percent of each final mark. Every year the same hierarchy emerged early on: investment bank and hedge fund veterans, often men, sliced through equations while others—including many women—sat frozen or spoke tentatively." Why? According to the article, it's because the women felt they had to choose between academic and social success. They held back their performances in class in order to be more dateable and look more attractive to the men. In other words, they Biffed. "I had no idea who, as a single woman, I was meant to be on campus," one student was quoted as saying. Were her priorities "purely professional, were they academic, were they to start dating someone?"

When a woman lacks her own internal compass, which is her connection to her pussy, she is lost at sea, no matter what the environment. Whether she is at Harvard, living in the Congo, traveling on the subway late at night, or coming out at a debutante ball, she has no inner sense of her inherent divinity or rightness.

The only thing that solves Biffing is a connection to pussy. A woman who owns her pussy owns her life. Knowing and owning the source of her feminine power is the only antidote to the crisis of confidence among women in the world today.

WOMEN BE ANGRY

When we Biff marriage or partnership, it's because we expect romantic love to deliver all of our most deeply held desires. In the process we overload ourselves—and our relationship—with hopes, dreams, and expectations. We believe it's our partner's job to fulfill us spiritually, romantically, sensually, and emotionally. Not only is it impossible for a single person to fulfill another on all of these levels, in adopting this belief we abandon our own sense of responsibility for our lives. Is it any surprise that half of all marriages end in divorce? The whole thing is a setup for failure from the start.

It is only since the Middle Ages that romantic love has been the basis for marriage at all. Prior to that, marriages were arranged for financial and social reasons. You might never have met the person you were to marry prior to walking down the aisle. Love was sometimes a happy accident, but it was not an expectation. The divorce rate has doubled since 1960, while the marriage rate has declined by 50 percent since 1970. A full 47 percent of adults are unmarried today. Of this group, 40 percent have been married before and are currently single, and 60 percent have never been married. The chance of a woman being a single mom is 50 percent, and one in three kids are being raised without a father. Of this group, only a third receive child support. Fifty percent of singles have not had a date in two years.

And yet women do not feel whole unless we are in a relationship.

As for the couples who stay married, the statistics are equally disheartening. Twenty percent of couples have sex 10 times a year or less. When it comes to sex drive, 30 percent of men and 50 percent of women report having none. When we do have sex, men have orgasms 75 percent of the time while women orgasm only 29 percent of the time. Perhaps unsurprisingly, infidelity is the number one cause of divorce.

I don't report these statistics to discourage you. To me they simply mean that the way we've done relationships up until now isn't working.

Teaching thousands and thousands of women over the last 20 years, I've discovered that one of the main reasons relationships break down is that the woman is disappointed in her partner. Her romantic expectations have not been met. What does she do when she realizes this? Does she graciously and generously teach her man how to please her? Does she lovingly educate him in the art of pleasing a woman?

Nope. She doesn't train, she complains.

Why would complaining—and ultimately, perhaps, dissolving the relationship—be her default? Because she has been programmed with a fairy-tale story line of what is "supposed" to happen. How her relationship is "supposed" to look and feel. So when the fairy tale doesn't work out as planned, she blames her man. She decides there's something wrong with him. She complains that he doesn't ask her what she wants—and that he wouldn't listen to the answers anyway. Meanwhile, the primary complaint men have is that they have no idea what their women want—and that their women aren't telling them, because we think they should already know!

What I know about men is that they really, truly live to make us happy. When we can find a kind way of telling them what we want, they are only too thrilled to comply. The problem is that we women are so deeply wounded by the masculine culture in which we've been raised that anger is what comes out first.

We live in an age when women have every right to be very, very angry. Our haircuts and dry cleaning are more expensive than men's, but we still get paid only 79 cents for every dollar a man makes. The medicines we're being given have primarily been tested on male bodies, rather than our bodies. We are not well represented in leadership positions, but overly represented in caretaker positions. In the corporate sector, the top leadership positions are held by men. As of this writing, only 2.4 percent of Fortune 500 CEOs are women, and out of 197 heads of state in the world, only 22 are women.

And what about the experiences we've each had on a personal level? I was groped and grabbed by men from the time I hit puberty. Women in my community have been date-raped, flashed, followed down streets in the dark of night, ignored when they spoke up, threatened, bullied, belittled, teased, catcalled, pressured into sex by bosses or colleagues, turned against when they've refused sex, and passed over in promotions because of their gender. You can't open a newspaper and not see stories of women and girls being sold for sexual slavery, being abducted and gang-raped by armies or even the policemen in their hometowns, being molested and sexually abused in their own families.

When a woman has been taught that the men in her life are not on her side, and that it's her job to accommodate them anyway, there is no way she can feel good about her interactions with them. She learns to submit to a balance of power that reverses the true power dynamic. She learns to act like she is the weaker party—even believe that to be true—when in fact, she is the stronger party. Remember, she is actually *the sun*. Any attempt to stuff herself down into the persona of helpless victim only makes her angrier.

One of the greatest difficulties a woman faces today is learning to take responsibility for her anger. This means to feel it, move it, Swamp it through her body—especially while being witnessed in sisterhood. Because no matter how justified and good her anger may be when righteously channeled, it can be problematic in the way it shows up in relationships. The only thing anger does in a relationship is destroy. Starting with the fact that it makes a woman feel awful about herself. Sure, it's not pleasant for him, but the real problem is that anger completely cuts her off from her own radiance. Without access to her innate resources, she feels even more powerless and frustrated. This frustration is felt as disapproval of her man. Meanwhile, if his woman is not feeling radiant, a man feels like a failure—just like we all feel cranky and depressed when we haven't seen the sun in a while.

When a woman learns that men are on her side, on the other hand, she recognizes that the way her man is (or isn't) showing up is a product of poor training, not bad intentions. Knowing that he's not trying to hurt or diminish her, she can relax. She is connected to her divine power source, so she is secure in the knowledge that there is always a way to get what she wants. When she is married to her radiance, there is always light on the path ahead.

RADIANCE TO THE RESCUE

Historically, women had to exchange sex for survival. Today, we are perfectly capable of putting food on our own tables and roofs over our own heads. In this way the balance of power has changed between men and women. We no longer need a man in order to live a healthy, happy life. In the process, the purpose of relationship has shifted from "food and shelter" to something else entirely.

A new paradigm of relationship is emerging. I like to think of it as *radiant relating*. This new relationship is a partnership that's created for the expressed purpose of taking one another higher. In a radiant relationship, his life gets exponentially better because she is in it, and her life gets exponentially better because he is in it. No longer an exchange based on need, this new relationship requires each person to consciously create pleasure for the other as an ongoing practice. Which means that each person has to approve of and appreciate the other, rather than be angry at them. Such an approach asks for a huge amount of self-examination, responsibility, and commitment. It's so easy to fall into the trap of blaming one another for what's missing.

In a radiant relationship, we are both active participants. Neither one of us can coast. We are each consciously looking to see how we can create some pleasure for ourselves and our partner, or communicate more and more transparently with our partner in order to know and be known even more deeply. The goal is to use the container of the relationship to take each other higher.

I have my own version of a radiant relationship. His name is Esteban, and he's been in my life more or less steadily for 10 years. Ours is not a partnership in any traditional sense. We come together, and then we go our separate ways. What we do when we are not with each other is not relevant. He is free to do what he wishes with whom he wishes, and so am I. There are no strings, no obligations. Each time we see each other, we both know that it might be the last—because neither one of us is interested in making a traditional commitment.

The foundation of our relationship is that we have very strong sexual chemistry. I see this man and I salivate. He is super-masculine: a martial artist who knows how to hold space for my feminine essence. Because I am such a powerful woman, it feels good to be with a man I can crash against, who won't crumble on encountering my intense passions. Esteban allows my wild, sensual animal to come out and play, and I don't have to hold anything back. I can be his queen and his whore in the same night. As I am someone who is in control in so many areas of my life, it is such a sweet pleasure to surrender and be a woman with him. Esteban knows me and loves me and admires me, and I feel the same about him. We really enjoy being with each other. And then, we both really enjoy our freedom. Our mutual understanding and our desire to make space for each other makes our "lovership" work.

When I first met Esteban, I told him that I was not interested in him as a boyfriend—just as a lover. I never felt like he was my "destination" the way I felt with Tiitus. We had both been married before and both had kids. For a while, we tried being boyfriend and girlfriend, but we felt kind of trapped and constricted in the roles. Such a traditional model didn't feel right for either one of us. We tried breaking up, but that wasn't right either. We liked each other too much to not want to be together—but we did not want to be exclusive.

At first it was hard for me to know he had other lovers. At first, he didn't tell me about it. He felt so wrong about that part of his nature that his instinct was to hide it from me to avoid losing me. I was more transparent with him; he knew I was seeing other men. When he finally revealed he was seeing other women, we nearly lost our relationship over it. It was hard for me to understand why he'd hidden his relationships. But it was also hard for me to face my truth: even though I didn't want a partner, my conditioning to be with one man exclusively remained very, very strong. I frowned on nonmonogamous relationships, even though I did not want a monogamous one.

Following this revelation, I broke up with Esteban for a year or so—and missed him terribly the whole time. I missed the incredible way he makes love to me. I missed talking to him. I missed the way he listens to me. The way he holds space for the highest and best part of me, even when I'm filled with doubt and fear. I missed that feeling of being able to relax into my feminine nature in his arms.

Then he showed up again. I was going through turbulence with my company, a very difficult period raising my daughter, and I had a loft under construction—all at the same time, and all by myself. One day I was walking down the street in my new neighborhood, and he was walking toward me. It was as if he was looking for me. When I asked him, he said he was. It seemed he knew I needed him, and the GPS had sent him out to find me. (I always look for synchronicities as a sign of being in the right place, at the right time, with the right man.)

When we ran into each other on the corner of Prince and Elizabeth Streets, I fell apart in his arms. It was as if we had just spoken the day before. I told him all of my heartbreak. He gathered me up, took me home, and made love to me. I felt so much better. He had come for me, found me, heard my story, and fucked me back to life. We have been lovers ever since.

There is a way that Esteban knows me, and knows what I need, better than anyone. I've had periods when I've wanted him to choose me, to the exclusion of other women. The conditioning to want the fairy-tale remains. In working this out for myself, I might push him away for a few months or longer. Yet I never end up choosing the fairy tale with anyone else. It's my particular relationship with Esteban that I want, and for this reason we always come back together. He listens to my stories, and I to his. He holds me with love and compassion, and I do the same for him.

We also have a lot of fun together. Occasionally we go to Miami for a few days. He might bring his guitar and play for me, and I might dance for him. We can have hours of lovemaking, beach time, and beautiful dinners. Then we separate, back to our lives. I enjoy inviting him to my lair, where I prepare for him as if he were my king and I, his courtesan. I pour a glass of his favorite wine or Pellegrino, and prepare a small tray of delicacies. I spend time preparing for him: bathing and dressing in my full courtesan gear, which might include hot lingerie and thigh-high boots, or a silky robe and delicately jeweled Manolos. I want to be absolutely radiant when he arrives. My radiance feeds me even more than it feeds him. I love inhabiting the space of my own turn-on. It brings out the best in me, allowing me to relax into my divinity through pleasure.

Our arrangement is certainly unconventional, but it works for me. For the past 10 years I have been on a tear: setting the SWA on its feet and finding my footing as a businesswoman; creating my core curriculum, teaching thousands of women, and building a team; raising my complicated, magnificent daughter and making a wonderful home for us. I have not wanted the complexity of bringing a man into our lives. I've wanted love and space and freedom and support and romance and great sex—all of which Esteban offers me.

Do I fantasize that one day Esteban and I will be together in the traditional sense? Sometimes I do. But deep in my soul I know that our connection would no longer be the radiance-generating machine that it is if we lived together and saw each other all the time. It's the wanting that keeps our connection alive. We were both married for a long time and are enjoying our freedom. We are meant to be lovers, and that is the frame that serves me best. It's always true desire that brings us together, which is more than most relationships can say. I continue to date other men, and I remain open to meeting someone who would be a good match for me in a more committed way. But right now, finding a partner is not my biggest priority. My priorities are my daughter and my work. Esteban makes both of those things better, and he does not distract me from my mission. It is actually a huge surprise to me how long we have been seeing each other. Why has our relationship been so healthy and long-lasting? Because we each serve each other's radiance.

Tuning In to What You Want

Radiant relationship is an exercise in options. The object is getting to the point of having choice: the choice to put our attention on a partner, or not. We no longer live in a world where we *have* to get married, or *have* to be in a relationship. While that feeling of urgency still lives inside of many women, the new paradigm of relationship is no longer all or nothing. We have a variety of choices available, and we are free to select the right one based simply on how radiant it makes us feel.

I am not interested in partnership at this time in my life, just like some people are not interested in investing the time and attention it takes to raise kids. But many of my students crave partnership, and I am happy to help them create it for themselves. I have assisted and supported thousands of successful partnerships over the past 20 years, even for women who had no idea that partnership was possible for them.

The entry point into radiant relationship is learning our own desires, following our pussy truth. This is not an easy road. It requires courage and a willingness to forge new tracks—tracks that work for us regardless of whether they look anything like a conventional relationship. When we really plug into our own desires, it turns out each of us wants something different. Some of us were born to get married and raise children in a wonderfully traditional sense. Some of us want kids, but no partner. Others want a partner, but no kids. Still others want lives of relative solitude. The object is to listen, to experiment, and to follow where your pussy leads. Very often, in order to do that, your ego has to get bumped out of the way. I know mine has been!

Putting a successful partnership in your orbit requires a lot of work. You have to give up certain aspects of your life. You are no longer flying solo; you have to consider someone else 24/7. When you're in a partnership, there are no time-outs or days off. Your emotional health and well-being are critical, not just for you but for your partner too. Partnership requires time and attention on the relationship, every day. Yet we get so much in return!

Every woman can write her own story of partnership, which is an ongoing adventure. For a woman to make any kind of progress in her life, especially in her relationship life, she has to love what *is*. This is not easy. I have had so many single women bemoan the fact that they are single and judge themselves as "wrong" for not being in a partnership. Judgment is like pouring sand straight in their gears. We cannot make any progress when we think what we have is wrong or bad. If I were to regard what I have with Esteban as wrong because it does not resemble the relationship my parents had, I would miss the point of my own creation. I have a very different life than my mother had, and a very different set of desires. It is both the luxury and the challenge of this age that I have the freedom and power to craft the perfect relationship for who I am, right now. In the process, relationship becomes a vehicle to get me more and more of what I truly desire—which right now means being able to focus all of my time on the work I love and raising my child, while still having wonderful soul-connected sex with

Esteban anytime I want. I imagine that when my daughter goes off to college I am going to want to go deeper with a man, and my relationships will change to accommodate that. That's what radiant relationship offers that a more traditional relationship structure does not: the flexibility to follow our desires in the moment, staying true to our pussy while honoring the partner (or partners) we engage with as both lovers and friends.

FINDING YOUR RADIANT WAY

Once a woman has located and owned her radiance, everything changes in terms of what she is looking for in a partnership. She has to find a man (or woman) who *amplifies* her radiance rather than diminishes it. Her desires and feelings have to be a priority for the relationship to be successful. Surprise, surprise, this is not something I was taught growing up. I learned that a woman is there to take care of her man and his needs—to make *him* feel great. None of my early partnerships were successful because I never made myself a priority. I followed the rules I'd been taught all my life, and I ended up feeling resentful and suffocated. Perhaps you have a similar story.

Owning our radiance is a continual and ongoing practice. We each must invest in stoking our own furnace, adding fuel to our radiant fire every single day. We cannot count on our partner to make us feel good; we must make that investment in ourselves. When we expect our partner to take care of all our needs, the relationship gets off balance. For example, if you ask your partner to give your body all the pleasure it requires (orgasms, massages, baths, pampering) you will just end up disappointed. Each of us has to make the investment in our own pleasure and make sure we have the attention we require to feel good about ourselves. If you keep your orbit at a high level, then anything your partner contributes is icing on your cake. For example, imagine scheduling your week to include daily Epsom salt baths and dance breaks, a handful of self-pleasuring sessions, quality time with turned-on women friends, and a massage and mani-pedi. Your radiance would be plugged in and turned on, before your partner even got involved. Anything he or she added to the mix would only enhance the bounty.

If you depend on your partner to provide all of this for you, the relationship can't help but go out of balance. Like anything that's out of balance, it will eventually die. The quality of your life is up to you. The greatest ongoing love affair you will ever have is the love affair you have with yourself. Having an amazing guy (or gal) by your side is just the gravy.

Too often I see women giving up their radiance to stay in an unsatisfying relationship or marriage. When Eve came to the School of Womanly Arts, she had been suffering low-grade depression for years. On the surface, she had everything a woman could ask for: a beautiful home, anesthesiologist husband, two beautiful kids. Yet she was miserable. She had spent her whole life trying to make her husband happy, in hopes that his happiness would lead to her own. Invisibly and imperceptibly she sank deeper and deeper into the cleanup/caretaker role, her life force draining from her body.

Her mother signed her up for Mastery, hoping to shake her out of her terrible downward spiral. After the first class weekend, Eve started to feel a bit more like herself again. She began to remember what "fun" felt like. Sleeping Beauty had begun to awaken.

That November we had a weekend class in Miami. Eve traveled there with another girlfriend and had a fabulous time. When an early snowfall threatened to impact her travel back to Buffalo, she watched her friend Sophie call her husband to inform him of the problem. He said, "Sophie, why don't you stay an extra day and get some spa treatments? Wait until the storm passes before you travel home."

Eve called her own husband, Howard, hoping for a similar response.

"Don't get any ideas," he said. "If you want to finish this program, you better get your ass home on time. I have been looking after the kids for three days and I am done!"

Eve went to the airport and had a hair-raising flight home, with so much turbulence that she was terrified and sick by the time she arrived. She took a taxi home, but Howard had not even cleared a path through the snow for her. The drifts were four feet high, and the taxi couldn't get close to her house. It was 3 A.M. when she finally dragged her suitcase over the snow banks and made it to the front door. She hauled herself inside and up the stairs to bed. Howard rolled over.

"You owe me a blow job, right now."

She got out of bed, went to the bathroom, and wept.

That was the moment she drew a line in the sand. She had reached the end of her marriage as she knew it. As she lay awake in the guest room, she realized that throughout her whole marriage, she'd been "earning her keep." She felt no better than a common prostitute, exchanging sex for food and shelter. Along the way, Howard had adopted her low opinion of herself. Something had to change. A subtle shift wasn't going to be enough—she had to do something radical. Howard would have to be willing to change, too, or the marriage would have to end.

It was time for them to do something radical together. It was time for them to start marching to the tune of pussy.

Eve had never, ever prioritized her pussy. She had married Howard because she thought he would be a good breadwinner and a good father to their children. She'd had only one other lover before she married Howard, and the sex was never that good with either of them. But at the time, she thought sex was unimportant. She thought she was supposed to pick a guy with earning potential, so that's what she did. Now she realized that ignoring her pussy had had terrible consequences for her life, her marriage, and her family. She was determined to set things right.

She realized that one of the reasons she was unhappy was that she and her husband had no chemistry. They'd been together for 10 years and had two children, but she'd never had a single orgasm. She was resentful that she was with someone who seemed to be much more interested in his work than in her and her needs. When Howard came home from work the next day, Eve was dressed in a sexy outfit; she poured him a glass of wine and sat in front of the fireplace with him.

"Look," she said, "we are both unhappy in this relationship. I have never had sexual pleasure with you. For all these years, you have never paid any attention to my pleasure. I have never had an orgasm my whole life. I cannot live like this anymore. We got married so early that I never really had a chance to experience dating, or learn about what I like, or explore who I am sensually. So here's what's going to happen—I am going to start prioritizing myself. I have made a decision that I am going to start dating other men. You are permitted to date me, but I am also going out with other men. I have to find myself, and my sexuality."

To her surprise, her husband was actually relieved to hear it. He wanted Eve to be happy; he just had no idea how to help her. With Eve willing to pursue her own happiness, he felt free—and excited at the thought of dating her again.

The two continued to share the same home and raise their kids, but she started going out on dates. On her next trip she met a man with whom she had great chemistry. She told him her whole story, and they became lovers. She kept her husband informed every step of the way. It was through her lover's kindness, gentleness, and patience that she was able to finally relax and experience an orgasm. They remained lovers for many months, and Eve was able to take the things she was learning about herself and lovemaking back to her husband. She taught him about her body, and she was able to open up to him more and more about her sensuality. Their sex life improved dramatically. Meanwhile, she and her husband had a special date night once a week, which added more fun and chemistry to their relationship.

Over the years since, they have continued to have an open relationship. Sometimes her husband has had a lover, with Eve's consent. Currently Eve has a lover, with her husband's full knowledge and agreement.

In this situation, both partners were willing to go off the traditional grid to figure out a structure that worked. It has required lots of communication and hard work to keep their partnership strong. But the effort has paid off, as they now have an alive, vital, intricate, intimate, growing, and changing partnership, which takes each of them higher. They have been married for 17 years, and continue to evolve. I am not implying that this couple has created a model that will work for others! This is a relationship that uniquely suits these two. It was the consequence of Eve locating her radiance and making her desires a priority. She took the very courageous step of transcending the cultural conditioning that was crushing her spirit to create a new kind of partnership that fed her soul.

When Jane, age 71, arrived at the SWA, she was wondering whether her marriage could work and was even considering divorce. Recently retired from a successful business career, her husband, Bob, had little sense of who he was, and he was feeling lost. They were not having fun. She was unsatisfied with their emotional connection and sex life, and was beginning to doubt whether that would ever change. For many years Jane had focused on her husband's problems. Being a family counselor, she believed that if she could help him, they could return to the love and connection they'd experienced in the first few years of their relationship. It never occurred to her to focus on *her* desires first. After enrolling in an SWA program, she took her attention off of fixing Bob—and put it directly on herself and her own pleasure. She threw herself into the practices: Bragging, Spring Cleaning, Swamping, Desire Lists, and Womantras. She focused on generating more pleasure for herself first, and only then invited Bob into it. She was shocked when he kept joining her. She was so surprised to learn that men not only want to but *love to* serve women's desires. Moreover, she discovered that a woman's capacity to receive is the key element in encouraging a man's giving. She learned that it's the pleasure she receives and appreciation she shares that motivates Bob. The more he feels seen, happy, and successful, the more he wants to please her so he can feel that way again. Today Jane only needs to ask for what she wants and Bob is happy to oblige—from running small errands to taking edgier steps like going to sensuality classes.

Jane also started listening more carefully to what Bob was saying. She used what she learned for her pleasure and his. For example, Bob would often tell her that she had "magic fingers." "Anywhere you touch me sends exciting feelings through my body," he told her. Because she listened, she now uses much more touch with him. It feels good to her, and makes him so happy. Their marriage has transformed from an exercise in frustration into an ongoing, ever-expanding adventure of radiant love.

Once we own our radiance, we must find ways to infuse that light into our partnerships. Otherwise the partnership must die. It is a man's job to amplify and encourage your turn-on, rather than diminish it. But it is *your* job to pursue your radiance at any cost. You cannot expect your partner to know what lights you up or turns you on. You have to do the research yourself.

Locating your radiance can be provocative. You might be living in the city and realize that you are more turned on by living in the country. You might have agreed with your parents and husband that it's probably time for you to have kids, but then find yourself unwilling to get off the pill. You might be in the middle of a divorce and then decide that you really, really want to stay married. Such a discovery may throw a curveball into your partner's or your family's life. But if that is what lights you up, everyone better jump on board and pack their bags. The sun is shining, and everyone needs that light.

From what I've seen over the years, men are mostly thrilled when their women stand proudly in their own radiance. But of course, there are those men (and women) with limited viewpoints who are not open to change or expansion. This can understandably be very frustrating for a woman who is just learning to prioritize her own inner glow. She will never find happiness with a partner who is interested in limiting her or diminishing her. Eventually she will have to decide whether to shrink herself down to fit her partner's comfort zone or to leave the relationship.

Maintaining Your Radiance

What lights us up and turns us on is ever-changing. The more demanding our lives are, the more rigorously we must attend to our pleasure. The year I wrote this book was challenging for me, because I had to add about 15 hours of writing time to my already full week. To keep my home fires burning, I also added on getting a weekly massage. I made sure I wore only hot-looking clothes to write in. I also made sure I moved my body a few times a week, going to S Factor, taking salsa lessons, SoulCycle, yoga, or working out with my trainer. The more I put out, the more I had to put in.

When writing in New York City, I made sure to light my favorite candle from the Hôtel Costes in Paris. When writing in Sag Harbor, I got up at 6:30 each morning to write at the beach for a few hours before the day began. Another great radiance-builder for me is to make sure I have sensual or sexual encounters every week. I have the luxury of living in New York City, where a school called OneTaste teaches a practice called Orgasmic Meditation. Orgasmic Meditation, or OM, is based on the stroking practice I learned when I was studying at More University. I have several OM partners—male friends who have studied this practice deeply and are always willing to have a stroking session with me. Between my OMs, my lover Esteban, and my self-pleasure sessions, I filled my tank with orgasm to fuel my soul—and this book!

Part of a woman's radiance comes from her ever-expanding sensual enjoyment of her body. I am a firm believer in the power of orgasm to fuel a woman's radiance. Whether you are single or married, it is your job to steer and guide your own sensual unfolding. You cannot leave your sensual fulfillment up to your husband or partner. You can have an orgasm any time you want with your own hand, a handheld showerhead, a Japanese Toto toilet, or an OM partner. It is unfair to blame the quality of your sex life on your partner. We can each do our part to expand the duration and intensity of our own orgasm. In doing so, we make ourselves much better partners for our lovers.

There are incredible teachers out there who have devoted their lives to the study of sensual education. If you prefer self-study, there are wonderful books you can read. (See the Further Resources section for some of my favorites.) The key is to *prioritize* and *invest in* your ever-expanding sensual life for the sake of feeding your own soul.

A radiant relationship is nothing more and nothing less than making the decision to serve your radiance as a priority in your relationship life. Does that seem selfish? I hope not. Keeping your own orbit high is the best way to be the most generous and loving you can be with your partner, lover, friends, family, and children.

Women have a tendency to think that sacrificing ourselves will serve the relationship, but the opposite is actually true. The more we plug into what turns us on, the more of our light we can shine on those we love.

Creating a radiant relationship is a journey. Just like any creation journey, the key is to get as clear as possible about what you want. Since we women are the source, we have to know where to shine our radiance. The dance of desire is a wonderful dialogue between you and that which is greater than you. The more we know what we want—the more we imagine the deliciousness of our desire—the more we actually attract it. The more a woman polishes her own altar and stokes the coals of her own brilliant radiant light, the more she can design her relationship life exactly the way she wants it.

FAVORITE FRAMES

Pleasure is a discipline that needs to be cultivated. There are three parts to any pleasurable experience: the planning, the execution, and the sharing of what I call Favorite Frames. The planning stage is the preparation. It includes anticipating the experience, creating the space, and organizing the who/what/where/when. Execution is the actual pleasurable experience itself, whether it's going to the movies, creating a sensual night for each other, or taking a trip to the beach. The last step—Favorite Frames—is one that too few of us have been taught. This is where we *reflect* on the experience that just happened and remember the highlights. That way, we not only get to enjoy the experience all over again, we get to digest the wonder and joy we just experienced.

Digesting a wonderful experience is super-important. When we don't digest, we remain "full." I don't have to tell you that when you've filled yourself up with a delicious meal, it's not comfortable to consume anything else. Pleasure is similar to food. It fuels us and feeds us. So when we fill up on pleasure, we get kind of stuffed. If we've hit our capacity and haven't yet digested, we might push away the next fun offer that comes our way. For example, after a wonderful session of lovemaking with your partner, it's super-sexy to describe to him the moments that turned you on the most. Then have him describe the moments that turned *him* on the most. It creates more intimacy and fun, and it also gives each of you a wonderful window into the other's experience. You might say, "It was so hot when you kissed me on the back of the neck, and then nibbled my ear. My pussy got so wet." Or, "When you threw me back on the bed, it was so unexpected. At first I was startled, but then it turned me on so much."

When we do not review our pleasurable experiences with others, we'll often find ourselves feeling really cranky. *Undigested goodness turns into negativity.* You've experienced it before—the hard landing after a really high peak experience. Most of us don't know why we feel that way, and we treat the crankiness as inevitable. But it doesn't have to be that way, and the answer is in sharing frames.

I often send a text the morning after a date, after a great party I attended or threw, or when a friend really shows up for me. Recently my friend Jeff came over and changed a lightbulb over the outdoor shower at my beach house. He'd noticed it needed changing a few weeks earlier, and I couldn't believe it when he showed up at my door with a new bulb. I made sure I texted him later to thank him for the experience. It extended and expanded the pleasure, and allowed for a soft landing back into our lives.

Homework: Sharing a Favorite Frame

Once you start sharing Favorite Frames, you won't want to stop! They're such fun, and they add pleasure to almost any situation. You can share a frame via text or e-mail, over the phone, or in person.

Over the next few days, keep an eye out for pleasurable experiences. They may be obvious ones, like a date or a party. Or they might be something more subtle, like a conversation with a colleague over lunch, or an act of service your man performed for you.

For each pleasurable experience you can point to, pick one or two of the highlights and share them with the person or people involved. Make sure to be very specific about the precise moment that was a favorite. Think of your frame as a snapshot, capturing a specific instance of pleasure. If you have multiple frames to share from the same experience, do them one at a time to get the greatest enjoyment and have the most impact.

For example, let's say you were doing frames of a great meal. It's far less powerful to say, "I loved our dinner!" than it would be to point out the specific things you loved. "The way you placed a small flower by each place setting was so beautiful and thoughtful." "I loved the simplicity of the fresh tomatoes and basil, with just a few drops of aged balsamic, and the most fragrant olive oil." See what I mean? Specifics create so much more turn-on and radiance.

Make a habit of doing Favorite Frames at least once a day, and you'll notice your enjoyment of your life will increase exponentially.

Radiant relationship is all about learning to live at a higher level of orbit, inside of our connection with another person. When we are plugged into what turns us on and lights us up, we are able to bring so much more connectivity and creativity to our relationship life. We not only inspire ourselves, but our radiance acts as a generator, igniting the light in our partners as well.

The whole purpose of this book is to reconnect women with our sense of power in the world in every aspect of our lives—including the world of relationships. Whether we realize it or not, we women spend a lot of our lives trying to "get ours." To get what we deserve, get what we want, get what we think we can't have. The feeling of scarcity that comes from our sense of lack is a result of thinking that the only way to be in relationship is by serving our partners. But when we reverse that idea and learn how to maintain our own radiance, the desperation to "get ours" falls away. In other words, we've finally learned *how* to get ours. As a result we feel powerful and confident in all areas of our life.

That sense of power and confidence translates not only into our one-on-one relationships with our partners, but—perhaps even more important—into our relationships with other women. This is the truth behind everything I teach. Once we have everything we've ever wanted, we can give generously to other women from our own surplus and take one another higher. Without supportive community, a woman can never hit the altitude she was born to inhabit. Humans are meant to live in community. We have simply lost our way inside of this patriarchal culture. When a woman learns to inhabit her own radiance, the first thing she wants to do is share it with another woman. I call this instinct Sister Goddess Activism, and it's at the heart of the movement I'll tell you about in the next chapter—the pussy-driven, radically radiant Pleasure Revolution.

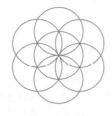

CHAPTER 9

THE PLEASURE REVOLUTION

*Open your heart, fling your hopes
high and set your dreams aloft.
I am here to hold your hand.*

— MAYA ANGELOU

When my daughter, Maggie, was born, I received lots of lovely cards and gifts. One card came from my cousin Eileen and her husband, Fred. There was a sweet illustration on the front that read, "A child is the root that binds a mother to her life." This card both fascinated and irritated me. I thought to myself, *Why do I need a child to bind me to my life? I already know what my life is about, and who I am.* So I put the card away.

But I did not throw it away.

Over the next few years, I found myself drawing it out every now and then to read that quote—still not entirely sure what it meant.

Now, 18 years later, I understand.

Some ancient part of me engaged the first time I took my newly born, crying Maggie in my arms. As I placed her on my breast and watched her settle in, I thought, *Oh my. I am in. I will do anything in my power to ease her tears and make her life good.*

What I noticed was that being a mother awakened parts of me that might never have awakened if I hadn't had her. Before Maggie, I did not know I was a force of nature in the body of a woman. Until it became my obligation to feed, clothe, and educate this child, I had no idea I was a talented entrepreneur, capable of creating a multimillion-dollar business out of a wild idea. I had no clue I was a powerful writer, a soul-changing educator, a world-transforming thought leader. In her iconic song, "I Am Woman," Helen Reddy sings that if she has to, she can do anything. Maggie Rose was my "have to."

For her, I would have done anything—including overcoming a tidal wave of my own perceived limitations.

In teaching thousands of students over the past two decades, I've discovered I am not alone. Trained as we have been by the PWC to think of others before ourselves, most of us would never even consider going the extra mile for our own pleasure, whether to achieve our own dreams or just because it felt good to do so.

But if there is another woman there who might benefit? Suddenly we find our motivation.

One of Grimms' fairy tales is called "The Handless Maiden." In this story, a miller makes a deal with the devil. He's so tired of being poor and not having enough food that he's willing to do anything. The bargain seems simple enough: The devil will make the man rich if the miller gives him everything in his backyard. Since the only thing the miller has in the backyard is a grove of apple trees, he readily agrees. The devil keeps his end of the bargain: The mill becomes very successful, and the impoverished miller becomes a wealthy man. It isn't until the devil returns to collect on his end of the bargain a few years later that the miller realizes what he's done. Unbeknownst to him, at the moment he'd made the deal with the devil, his beautiful daughter had been playing among the apple trees in the backyard.

Devastated, the miller begs the devil to leave his daughter behind. The devil relents, saying, "If you cut off her hands and give them to me, I will leave her with you." The miller eagerly agrees; he chops off his own daughter's hands to keep her at home with him.

The miller's daughter is overwhelmed with pain and betrayal. She runs away and wanders for days. Overcome by hunger, she wanders the orchard of the king's castle looking for a bit of fruit to eat. There she encounters the prince—who falls in love with her beauty and her helplessness. He marries her and has a pair of silver hands crafted for his new wife.

When she is happily pregnant, the prince leaves to go to war. In his absence, the princess gives birth to their child and sends a message to the prince announcing the joyous news. But the devil—still angry over losing the young woman—interferes with the message; the prince receives word that the princess has given birth but that the child is a changeling. The prince writes back that she should care for the child anyway. Again, the devil intercepts the message, replacing it with an order for the princess and the child to be killed.

Terrified, the princess runs away from the castle with the baby strapped to her back. After many hours of walking, she comes to a stream. As she leans over to get a drink, the baby slides off her back and into the water. The princess plunges her handless arms into the stream, desperate to save her drowning baby. To her amazement, her hands grow back immediately, allowing her to rescue her child—and in so doing, rescue herself.

INTRODUCING SISTER GODDESS ACTIVISM

I, like many women, was that handless maiden. I had no idea how powerful I was until my daughter was born. In the amazing opportunity of raising her, *I raised myself.* I found my voice as a leader. I began to take the greatest creative risks of my life, and to succeed beyond my dreams. I could not—would not—have had the confidence in myself to do what I have done had I not been doing it on behalf of my girl.

When a woman takes her pleasure-filled attention and places it on another woman, the result is that both get to go higher than they ever could have alone.

It takes another woman to reflect back our greatness to ourselves. Take the experience of giving birth. There's always a moment where the contractions are so great that the laboring woman says, "I can't! It's too much. I can't take the pain. Get me out of here!" What she needs at that moment is not a drug, or a knight in shining armor, or any other sort of rescue. She needs another woman who has been through it before to say, "I know it fucking hurts, but you can do it! You *so* got this." Somehow, through the support of another woman, we find the resources within ourselves to persevere. We can step into our power in a way that re-creates our understanding of who we are and what we are capable of. We also learn that the "Oh, no, I can't" comes just moments before the baby (real or metaphoric) is placed in our arms.

An initiated woman is a woman who has been through this same process before. Who once believed herself too small for the task at hand, but who—through the grace of *another* woman's attention, inspiration, love, and reflection—broke through to a new level of turn-on and power. A woman who other women stood for, until she could plug back into her own turn-on and power.

A woman I call a Sister Goddess Activist.

Sister Goddess Activism (SGA) locks in when another woman needs something that we have to give. In the process of offering her something she requires, we find a strength and power that we did not know we possessed. Both of us become the women we were meant to be, together.

Sister Goddess Activism starts with standing strongly for our own radiance, which allows another woman to stand for hers. It requires us to love ourselves for no good reason, except that we can. In the process, we spread the virulent condition of self-love to every woman and girl we encounter. SGA means standing powerfully in our connection to our pussy, and being willing to risk speaking our pussy truth. As uncomfortable as it might be, we know our action will take someone else higher—so it's well worth the risk.

Luckily, we do not have to have our shit together to participate in SGA. Not at all. The only requirement is that we've committed ourselves to standing for our radiance. Once we make that pledge, the Great Pussy in the Sky guides us toward exactly the woman who requires our unique brand of inspiration. What she will need from us is the very thing we doubt the most in ourselves. She might need to be inspired to ask for a raise at work—something we ourselves would be scared to do. But we can see the value in *her* that we could not see in ourselves. The result is a magical alchemy: Somehow we find ourselves powering up that part of us in ways we would not have been capable of before. And we do it so we can model it on her behalf.

Your Desires Set Me Free

We need such models, because there is a way in which every woman in our culture is a handless maiden.

We have all been taught that it is our birthright to be handless and helpless. We cannot possibly inhabit our radiance if we have no idea what it is, what it feels like, and what it means. And if we have not stepped into our radiance, we have not stepped into our power.

At the same time, we all have an innate willingness to do just about anything to save or help another. The handless princess was powerless—until her baby's life was at risk. This fable points to the unfortunate truth that a woman will not step into the fullness of her power for herself alone. In reality, we *can't*—because until our power is required by another, *we do not know that we have it in us.* We can't boldly go where no woman has gone before, because we don't know that territory exists until we are forced to go beyond our limitations on behalf of another.

That we women require one another to achieve our own innate greatness is itself extraordinary and wonderful. It means that the places where I doubt myself the most are my opportunities to connect with my greatness. Together is the only way for any of us to hit our maximum potential, to live into the deepest corners of our dreams and desires. To step boldly into our radiance and inspire other women by being a model of turn-on. It's the most wonderful construct: your desires will set me free, and mine will set *you* free. Not only does it turn out that there is more than enough of everything for all of us to get what we want, but our ability to get everything we desire, and then some, actually *hinges* on our participation in Sister Goddess Activism. Helping another woman get into her highest orbit is the fastest way for us to get into ours.

When we choose to step into SGA, we are taking responsibility for someone else's pleasure. Which is like paying it forward to the GPS—who always gives it right back to us a thousandfold. Even though we may not choose activism in order to get something, we actually *do* get rewarded, not just by the pleasure of the act itself but by becoming even more irresistibly able to attract our own desires.

SISTERHOOD AS SALVATION

Born into the Patriarchal World Culture, we women don't realize we are only partially living the lives we were destined for. We have been indoctrinated not to recognize—and thus, not to call forth—the native power that is our birthright. It is only when a woman stands fiercely for another human being's freedom that she experiences the fullness of her power. We can see this in the women who came forward at the end of the 19th century to abolish slavery. Harriet Tubman, an escaped African-American slave, did not simply make her way to the North and settle in for a comfortable life. She understood that slavery is as much a mind-set as it is a situation. To free herself internally, she devoted the rest of her life to freeing others.

She once said, "I freed a thousand slaves. I could have freed a thousand more if they only knew they were slaves." She understood that even when literal freedom is granted, it may not mean the former slave is truly free. There is an internal game change that has to take place. One way to make this internal shift is to become an activist on behalf of others. When you change your perception of yourself from slave to activist, you transform from victim to heroine.

If only more women understood that we, too, are slaves.

That we are enslaved to the patriarchy.

That our negative thoughts are not the truth.

That we are not everything we've been indoctrinated to believe we are: Unimportant. Valueless. Clueless. Fat. Old. Losers. Incapable.

We have no idea that these perceived limitations are not real.

We have no idea what our potential is.

We have no idea of the scope and reach of the power of our desires.

We have no idea that our feminine perspective is life-changing for those whose lives we touch.

No idea that we bring life and light to every situation and circumstance.

No idea that our much-disparaged pussies will not lead us down the path to hell—but rather, down the path to freedom.

No idea that we are the embodiment of the divine on earth.

And most important, no idea that *sisterhood is our salvation.*

That we must stand for one another in order to become the heroines of our own lives.

This book—and the work of my entire life—is promoting a new type of activism. This activism goes beyond the boundaries of feminism as we've understood it. It is based not in anger and indignation, but in joy and pleasure. It's an activism that is undertaken by women, for women. It's about taking other women higher in order to take *ourselves* higher. It incorporates spirituality, social justice, radiant turn-on, and reverence for nature. It focuses beyond the individual; it thinks globally. It welcomes women of every religion and every background joining together in feminine connection, inclusion, and spirituality. This revolution is here to take the world to a new level of turn-on.

This belief system is the Pleasure Revolution. And it starts with SGA.

For example, Sister Goddess Denise was an accountant—an extremely *under-earning* accountant. She was making $35,000 as the business manager for an electrical company when she came into the SWA. She wanted to start her own business but didn't feel successful or powerful enough to step into the role of leader and coach. Deep in her heart she thought she would be really good at it, but her doubt was way bigger than her dreams.

At the School she made a lot of Sister Goddess girlfriends. With their help, Denise decided to launch a website offering her financial services. One of the women in the group, Sister Goddess Dara, was in the process of opening a dance and yoga studio in Brooklyn. She wanted Denise to help with some of the bookkeeping. When she looked at Denise's website, however, she was shocked. Denise had created a website that made her look like an average accountant, filled with pictures of boring people in suits and totally lacking sex appeal. Denise's nickname at the SWA had been "Sexy Money." Dara told her she needed a new photo shoot and a new energy. After a lot of protesting, Denise finally had a photo shoot and brought more of her pussy truth onto the website. Soon thereafter, she had her first $8,000 month. She now has a thriving business, not just doing accounting but teaching online courses on money for women.

Dara stood for the radiant version of Denise she knew from the SWA—not letting her off the hook just because her stodgy website was more comfortable for Denise. Sister Goddess Activism is about inspiring one another out of our comfort zone, so we have a chance to hit our *desire* zone. Dara's unflagging belief in Denise's power sent both of them into a higher level of orbit. Denise got the business she wanted and deserved, and Dara got the radiant accountant she needed to help launch her studio. This mutual benefit is what SGA is all about.

UNLEARNING THE RULES

Now comes the difficult part: unlearning what we've learned about woman-to-woman relating. Because the norms of the PWC do not teach us to embrace sisterhood. On the contrary, we women have been taught that we are not to be trusted, not to be counted on, and not to be brought in close. We've been taught to believe that women are backbiting, envious, catty, emotionally unstable, hysterical, premenstrual, and unreasonable. We have been taught that, given the chance, women will take each other down. If you turn your back for a second, she'll steal your job or your man! If you let her get close, she'll use you for social climbing! If you tell her your good ideas, she'll take credit for your work! She'll put you down in front of others to make herself look good! If she doesn't betray you right away, she certainly will eventually.

Whoa. No wonder we all feel so suspicious and disconnected from one another.

Perhaps the worst consequence of this belief system is that we end up unable to connect to other women in joy, radiance, and pleasure. If we want connection with other women, we must get it via our mutual victimization. We end up able to communicate only about the negatives in our lives. We are likely to talk about what kind of flu bug we just had, or bitch about our boss, or complain about how our husband forgot our birthday again. But we don't dare reveal anything *good* about ourselves, or our lives. We would never share about the great sex we just had with our hot boyfriend, or how much we love our job and how incredibly well-paid we are. Why? *We don't want other women to feel bad.* We assume that there isn't enough good to go around, so our radiance is a threat to other women. We don't want her to hate us for having a great life, so we stay focused on everything that's going wrong. To relate with other women, we must connect around our bad luck, mistreatment, and despair. Bad news is our entry point; we have absolutely no shame about leading with the negative. But to start with the spectacular news of our lives? We cringe.

This kind of cultural agreement is another form of enslavement. It binds us to negativity, instead of our potential. When a woman is taught by her culture to only communicate about the negative, she begins to place "positive value" in the negative. It becomes our negative experiences that buy us access into relationship with other women. With Sister Goddess Activism, the new style of pleasurable relating with other women is to brag about, revel in, and celebrate the wonderful things that we have created in our lives. Pleasurable relating reeducates a woman that her achievements have value—not only to herself but to other women. They give her an opportunity for a new kind of bonding. Women celebrating women becomes a new way of relating. And when you have a community of practice in which to brag, you end up inspiring others to take bold action in their lives. Bragging is, itself, a form of activism on many different levels.

What SGA Is Not

Sister Goddess Activism turns many more of our cultural norms on their head. Most of us have been taught that when a suffering or sad woman reaches out to us, she's likely to cling like a needy vine, sucking our very life away. But in SGA, we continually turn her back on to herself. The agreement is that we simply take a stand for her: encouraging and inspiring her to follow her own pussy, rather than ours. We never become the *source* of her power.

A Sister Goddess Activist is not a coach, a therapist, or a social worker. It's not our job to tell her what to do; oftentimes we may not even address the "problem" she is having. We are there to share some of our radiance in order to tune her back in to her own pleasure channel. For example, say the woman you encounter does not have a man to date. It's not your job to give her dating advice or to tell her what she's doing wrong. And it's certainly not your job to find her a man to date! You are simply holding up a mirror so she can tap into her own radiance. After all, the whole goal of SGA is to inspire a woman to turn back on. Each of us acts like a candle, lighting other women's candles until our whole world is illuminated.

As Sister Goddesses, we also reject the norm that says we need to join another woman's pity party. The PWC has taught us that being a good friend means to commiserate with another woman's lack. Sister Goddess Activism instructs us to do the opposite. Instead of saying, "Oh you poor thing! I'm in the same boat," we say, "Got it. Hear you, feel you. And guess what? Yes you *can* do it, and you're *going* to. I am standing for you, sister. We're going to make this shit happen."

When a woman has a problem or obstacle, our culture commonly tells her she needs to do something to fix *herself.* Like get another degree, or go to therapy, or call her psychic. She gets redirected away from the problem and down some big rabbit hole. Sister Goddess Activism puts the focus on getting her turned on before anything else. This sometimes means that you have to challenge her, just like Ama-no-Uzume challenged Amaterasu. She did not give the abused goddess a shoulder to cry on—she gave her a pussy party. This challenged Amaterasu to remember who she was: a divine woman capable of continual creation and re-creation. In the same way, SGA demands to see a woman's divinity, rather than agreeing with her that it is inaccessible or gone. Rather than both parties descending to the depths of hell together as a way of soothing each other (which is what the PWC teaches us to do), SGA throws down the pussy gauntlet and gives both women a chance to step into a new aspect of their power.

Sometimes the recipient is too deep inside the PWC to even catch a whiff of her own pussy perfume. She may insist, no matter what, that life is wretched and horrible and unsalvageable. No problem: The Activist knows this is an ideal time to Swamp. To invite her sister to pour her grief through her own body. To scream, rage, cry, pound pillows, chop down trees—whatever it takes to move it through.

If after a good Swamp the woman still cannot summon the ability to change paradigms and see her own magnificence, there is one fail-safe way to get her there.

Ready?

It's to have *her* perform an act of SGA for a woman who is in a similar boat. It's to present her with a woman who requires *her* turn-on, to power up her own. When another woman is in need, we will find reserves within ourselves that we could not have imagined even existed.

Truth: I could not have started the School of Womanly Arts for myself. But I could do it for Maggie. I could do it for *you* . . . for *them* . . . for all the women in the world who will never, ever have a chance to have a woman stand for them. I did not have to find a way to rise. I simply fucking *rose*.

I would not be who I am today without this community of womanhood, of which you are now an essential part.

We need each other. But it is not the neediness of old; it is not the neediness of dependence and desperation. It is not the neediness of mutual victimization. I *need* you to be as big, blazing, and radiant as you can possibly be. Because the more of your legendary light you step into, the more of mine I can inhabit and embody. By standing in my own sacred radiance, I open up room for you to stand in yours—beyond the parameters of what you or I can imagine.

When I set my pussy free, somewhere in this world I set other pussies free.

LIFE AT ALTITUDE

When you stand for a woman this way, or are stood for in this way, the result is a collision of emotions that is difficult to describe. When you stand for her to find the resources within herself, you are challenging her to connect with the best and brightest and most spiritually alive aspects of herself. You are showing her that she can hold hands with her divinity—that she already knows how. It is so moving to witness, because you know what it's costing her to do that. It is costing her lifelong belief in her own victimization. It's costing her the convictions she's held since childhood that she is unworthy or less than. It's costing her that deep, abiding sense that she is spiritually alone and unloved. Seeing your belief in her potential, she must give up all the things that keep her small yet feel like safety to her. As I mentioned in the first chapter, Diane von Furstenberg would have to give up feeling like a loser. Gayle King would have to give up feeling fat. Sheryl Sandberg would have to give up feeling like a fraud. I cannot emphasize enough how difficult this shift can be. For all these things feel like *home* to a woman. She has to give up what's familiar in exchange for the turn-on she secretly hopes is available.

She will want to revert to her old ways. Only inside of a framework of Sister Goddess Activism—only when witnessed, inspired, and encouraged by other women—will she have the bravery to keep stepping forward. Watching a woman make this transition is so heartbreakingly beautiful. It's one of the greatest joys I know, to witness her as she experiences, often for the first time, that she is more—so much more—than she thought she was.

All it takes is one decision: the decision to trust her pussy and her turn-on above all other values.

And a Sister Goddess who reminds her that she doesn't need anyone to grant her light, because she is the light.

At the moment she really gets that, there are tears, but they are not like the tears of old. There is emotion, but it's not sad. In truth it's a little bit shocking.

"You mean I am the Goddess?! After a whole life of feeling like a persona non grata?"

This particular combination of spine-tingling emotions—being shocked and moved and touched by your own magnificence—doesn't come from any other experience that I know of.

It takes no courage at all to feel pathetic; it's so easy to do. The thing that takes courage is to choose radiance when you're not feeling it. And to help someone else choose hers. It takes a community of turned-on, radiant sisterhood to set this stage. It is my hope that everyone reading this book will have access to such a community, and soon. (See the Further Resources section at the back of the book for a start.) I believe we can all live to see a world of Sister Goddesses within our lifetimes. Women who are turned-on and standing in our radiance—when we walk down the street, tend our children, love our men, look into the eyes of a sister, make our way to work. It does not require a system or a doctrine. All it requires is one woman standing for her own radiance, and then standing for the radiance of another woman. And then, for the radiance of all women.

We all have access to it. We just have to get to the altitude where we can see it.

PLEASURE SLAVE DRIVER

We are always opening doors for others, whether we know it or not. We do it simply by shining our radiant light on the world. Your radiance never goes unnoticed. It is never *not* inspiring. It is always profoundly valuable. Yet we all have blind spots, areas in our lives where we are not able to step into the full power that we possess. That's where SGA comes in. When I can't see my power, I don't have to worry. There is another Sister Goddess who sees it for me. She can serve as an inspiration and placeholder until that part of me catches up.

A few years ago, a beloved friend and student, Ayodele, was taking one of our advanced courses. Her ass was dragging very low to the ground. She had just been through a series of devastating losses. First, her mother died after a protracted illness. Then her best friend, a young woman named Sonia, died of cancer. The final crushing loss was the sudden death of her mentor and friend—Barbara Ann Teer, the founder of the National Black Theatre.

When a woman is having a particularly difficult time in her life, she may need one-on-one support. I have a special role for my more advanced students, which I call Pleasure Slave Driver. This is where one student will agree to "pleasure slave drive" another, ensuring that the first woman builds enough pleasure into her life to keep her flying at a high altitude. The idea is for the Pleasure Slave Driver to press her, very nearly against her will, to hold the space of her own radiance. Because even though we don't usually live this way, it *is* possible to be radiant when you are grieving, as well as when you are celebrating. The key is to tune your instrument to the octave that your soul is currently singing.

Ayo had been grieving these losses for so long that low-level grief was the octave she was most comfortable playing in. But Ayo knew she was not living up to the potential of her brightest light. Her desires were starting to break through her grief—like the desire to date after 30 years alone. She started to feel scared, realizing that she'd never consistently lived in her brightest light. She'd had fits and starts of brightness after she landed in the Sister Goddess community, but it was not enough to keep her own engine gassed.

Sarah volunteered to be Ayo's slave driver, knowing how fun it would be to use her pleasure-filled attention to take another sister higher. Every day Sarah would wake up and meditate and see what pleasurable ideas bubbled to the surface on Ayo's behalf. She found that tapping into her deepest intuition and knowing resulted in the most remarkable ideas.

She ordered Ayo to create an altar to herself. She felt that Ayo was a queen and had merely forgotten. If you don't remember you're a queen, it's really hard to date. "It was flat-out shocking for her to do it," Sarah told me. "But she went for it. The next time we were in class, she bragged about the experience. She had taken my idea, blown it up into this beautiful thing, creating a gorgeous poem to herself and creating the most elaborate altar. It was stunning. I gave her a mustard seed, and she made this thing of beauty."

Today, Ayo is engaged to be married for the first time, at age 69. She kept telling Sarah, "You did this, Sarah, you did this!" But all Sarah did was remind Ayo that she had the Goddess inside. She stood as a mirror for Ayo's magnificence, reflecting her beauty back to her, which allowed Ayo to go into the world with a greater sense of self. Ayo didn't have to go after that wonderful man; she simply drew him in.

I asked Sarah how providing Sister Goddess Activism has impacted her personally.

"In order to stand for another woman, you have to first stand for yourself," Sarah told me. "You must play big in your life, so the other woman can be inspired by you. We are taught to care for others, but activism teaches you to stand for yourself first—and to give from your overflow."

Overflow. It's not an easy concept to describe to a woman who has not tapped into her pussy. But a woman who is connected to her radiance and is continually investing in her pleasure is no longer desperate or needy or empty. Her tank is full. So full, in fact, that she has to begin to do something with all the extra love she feels inside. That's when she knows it's time for her to perform a random act of SGA. Only once a woman is filled up does she have something of value to offer. Women have been in a state of emptiness for so, so long. Finding our radiance means that we suddenly have energy to spare. The best way to use that energy is on behalf of another woman, because it takes all of us higher.

TEAM ACTIVISM

Activism can be especially powerful when we get knocked resoundingly on our ass. When we get an unexpected gift from the Great Pussy in the Sky, like a diagnosis of cancer. When my student Elvira turned 60, she received such a diagnosis. She'd had cancer 17 years earlier, when she was newly divorced with two small children and a new job. Back then she'd toughed it out and gotten through it on her own, fueled by grit and determination not to abandon her kids.

This time around, she was a Sister Goddess. She told her community of Sister Goddess friends what was happening and asked for their support and help. She knew she could not do it by herself this time. Her gang of women was amazing. She never went alone to a doctor's appointment. The women who went with her were nutritionists, breast cancer survivors, and doctors—all asking the questions she herself was too scared to ask. Her surgeon finally asked her, "Who are you? And who are all these people?" Elvira proceeded to educate her surgeon about sisterhood.

Together they practiced the Tools: Dance Breaks, Spring Cleaning, healing circles, whatever it took. Someone even made T-shirts that said "Team Elvira." The surgery team met Elvira's Sister Goddesses the day of her surgery. Right before they put her under, the surgeon and plastic surgeon lifted their gowns to reveal they were wearing "Team Elvira" T-shirts!

The Sister Goddesses made sure that someone was sitting with Elvira's daughter in the waiting room during the surgery. When Elvira woke up, the first faces she saw were those of her daughter and five Sister Goddesses. When she returned home, the Sister Goddesses had organized themselves in shifts so there were always at least two at her home, round the clock. They brought food, cleaned the house, walked the dog, helped her to the bathroom, and gave her daughter a much-needed night off.

Her first experience with cancer was filled with fear. She was so afraid. So scared for herself and her daughters. This second experience with cancer was entirely different. She knew that her sisters had her back, no matter what happened. She knew that if she had attracted this level of love and support, she could do anything—even cure herself of cancer. Sisterhood gives us the strength to believe in the best and brightest aspects of ourselves and to connect deeply to our power.

Becoming an SG Activist

So how do you begin to be a Sister Goddess Activist? How do you take the messages you've gotten that tell you women are untrustworthy and turn them on their head? How do you fill yourself up enough that you are able to fight for pleasure and meaning on behalf of another woman? The answer is simple. You start with your pussy. You start by listening to what she wants and giving her what she needs. You prioritize your own self-care in a world that tells you that your experience doesn't matter. You fill up on pleasure, radiance, and turn-on until you have more than you need—and the result is a natural outpouring of love toward your sisters.

This is why this chapter comes at the end of this book rather than at the beginning. Until you are filled up with your own radiance, there is no way to shine that radiance onto the world. Sister Goddess Activism would not even occur to a woman who was not plugged into her turn-on. Over-giving and martyrdom are not Activism. Although they are states that feel incredibly familiar to women, they are the antithesis of SGA. Activism feels joyful; it feels fun. You have to be feeling pretty fine about yourself in order to play.

The requirements to become a Sister Goddess Activist are simple:

- You realize that your life is a gift, and you are oh-so-grateful to the GPS to be alive.

- You live in the land of possibilities, knowing every single one of your desires is on its way to you—under grace and in perfect ways.

- You notice that wonderful things are always happening to you, and you are willing and able to brag about your life at any moment.

- You know how to manage your own garbage. You don't blame others when things don't seem to go your way; you immediately grab the Tools of Swamping or Spring Cleaning to get back in balance.

- You are sensually alive and engaged. Your pussy is turned on. You stand in your powerful radiance every single day.

- You have a strong Sister Goddess community surrounding you, with whom you practice the Tools and Arts daily.

A Sister Goddess knows that every single step in her story line has been created of her, by her, and for her. She knows that she is no one's victim. She has rejected the cultural pull toward commiseration and victimhood. She replaces these habits with the unshakable sense that she, herself, has called in every circumstance in her life for the purpose of taking her higher. She remembers that, through rupture, the Goddess is remaking her into the woman she was born to become. She knows, deep inside herself, that there is an inherent rightness, an inherent perfection to everything and everyone. She is not thrown off her spiritual path when some devastation happens to her or to another Sister Goddess. She lives in the truth that every moment is a gift, and every stroke is a chance to go higher.

Homework: Sister Goddess Activism

Celebrate a woman in your life today. Your goal is to take her higher. Tell her how much she means to you in person or on the phone, or write her a letter of appreciation and gratitude. Teach her how to brag with you. Ask her what she wants and find out how you can be her wingwoman.

Imagine a world where every woman takes another woman higher. Imagine a world where we see "sister" every time we look into another woman's eyes. We can do this. We *can* make this change in our lifetime. One pussy at a time.

OUR PROMISE TO THE WORLD

When a woman knows these truths to be self-evident, she is ready to take her show on the road. She is ready to be of service to the world as a Sister Goddess Activist. Instead of following the old, worn-out story that women will betray and hurt one another, a Sister Goddess promises to see "sister" every time she looks into another woman's eyes. She knows that no matter if she is under a burka in Afghanistan, sitting in a lounge chair at the Beverly Hills Hotel, crawling through the rubble of a recent bombing in Syria, setting her foot on a red carpet in Cannes, cleaning a bathroom, or running a board meeting at a Fortune 500 company—every woman on this planet is her sister, and every woman on this planet is the Goddess.

She is always practicing an elevation of consciousness. She sees taking other people higher as a form of delicious entertainment—as both a living prayer and a badass lifestyle. She likes inspiring men, women, and children into a higher state of awareness and appreciation with the attention she places on them. She is a radiant, embodied woman who makes the investment to enjoy every step of her journey. Flirtation is her middle name. As a consequence, she inspires others through the pleasure that she takes in herself.

With Sister Goddess Activism, all the advantages of the feminine are returned to the culture from which they were taken, 5,000 years after the patriarchy began to dominate. As a result, the consciousness of the culture elevates and evolves. For example, the current paradigm of justice says, "An eye for an eye, and a tooth for a tooth." When something bad happens, we are taught to exact revenge. The feminine paradigm is very different. When something bad happens, we first reach for grieving. For *feeling*. For *connection*. Then we ask the question, "What is needed to take this higher?"

We are the breakout generations. We are each the women leaders who were born here, born now, inside of a culture that desperately requires the leadership and viewpoints of the feminine. *Your voice matters*. This world needs your voice so that it can transform and begin to rebalance the masculine and feminine energies. The world is hungry for new ideas, and the voice of the radiant feminine is the voice of transformation in our lifetime. Women are the greatest untapped natural resource on this planet.

We women free ourselves when we free one another. That is the way of Sister Goddess Activism. The way of pussy. And the way of the future.

I'd like to leave you with a poem that one of my students, Sister Goddess Christine White, wrote as a pledge to support the Pleasure Revolution.

Ready for the world, hot, throbbing, and wet.
My pleasures are treasures. My desires are met.
Sister Goddesses together, what we want, we get.
Our community is truly ecstasy in the flesh!
And I'll never forget that Pussy knows best
'Cause when a woman's turned on
The whole world is blessed!

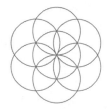

AFTERWORD

I cannot even describe the gratitude that I feel toward you for having gotten this far into *Pussy*.

You are brave and astonishing.

From the time I was a small girl, I promised to set the patriarchal problems I perceived to rights in my lifetime. Ever since, I have been on the adventure of creating this book. It's my doctoral thesis, my chef d'oeuvre, my love letter to the world that we are all privileged to live in.

It is my greatest wish that this book make it into the hands of women everywhere. Women of every shape and size, every possible life experience, every nook and cranny of our culture. For if there is anything I have learned in my role as Mama Gena it's that, as different as we seem, we are all the same. We are all women. We are all radiant, exceptional, divine. We all rapture, rupture, and rapture again.

In other words, we are all *pussy*.

I always knew, deep inside myself, that despite the evidence, women are not "fucked up." The world might be out of balance, and the consequence of that imbalance might skew our perspectives and experiences, but the nature of each human being is truly and essentially divine.

Each of us longs to find a way to make sense of the life we have been given. At this particular moment, our world is flooded with high priests- and priestesses-in-the-making. We're flooded with feminine leaders looking for the best way to inhabit their mission, flooded with visionaries waiting for the moment to step into the power they have been cultivating. It is my desire that this book serve as fuel to feed those voices. That it inspire the creative action our world so desperately requires in order to evolve and heal.

My job is to initiate. To give women the opportunity to forfeit victimization. To hand them the arts and tools required to become the hot and sexy heroines of their own life stories. So that they can initiate others, and return our world to its rightful balance.

And oh, what a journey! Life with a turned-on pussy is an adventure worth living for.

Your desires will take you places you could never have dreamed. You will find talents you never knew you possessed, and you will create opportunities that will continually astonish and amaze you.

Yes, *you*. You are that powerful and splendid.

With my one small life, I have had the opportunity to love and be loved oh-so-very deeply; to contribute devoutly and mightily; to live my extraordinary range of gifts and talents; and to release millions of women to live theirs.

My wish for you?

The same, and then some.

This is what I want you to know:

You are not alone.

You are of such inestimable value.

Whatever difficulties, obstacles or seemingly insurmountable challenges are choking your life force, they are not permanent, there is a way around, and this book will help you by connecting you to the divinity that has always been inside of you.

This book is your road map. I made it for you to light your way.

But *you* must take the step.

So- how will you re-consecrate your altar today? Some fresh flowers on your bedside table? An Epsom salt bath?

How will you relate to your husband differently? Will your inner courtesan ask him for what you want?

Who will you give a copy of this book to, in order to expand your circle of sisterhood? Will you start a woman's group and practice the exercises?

Will you pick up the phone and teach a girlfriend how to do a holy trinity with you?

How will you celebrate your womanhood at dinner tonight, blazing a trail for your daughter to celebrate hers?

How will you bless yourself with your own approval, today, and every day?

Go on then. Take that turned-on pussy out for a spin and set the world on fire with your magnificent desire. Live that legend, sister. I will be here, holding your hand.

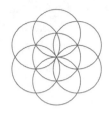

APPENDIX

The Womanly Tools and Arts

Throughout this book, I've referred to the Womanly Tools and Arts. The Arts were covered in depth in my first book, *Mama Gena's School of Womanly Arts*. The Tools have been developed more recently and are at the core of what I teach in the School of Womanly Arts Mastery program. Here's a little overview of each of these highly useful techniques and technologies. For a deeper dive with any of the Arts, pick up a copy of the earlier book. If you want to get down and dirty with the Tools, why not join us at our next Mastery program?

THE WOMANLY ARTS

1. *The Womanly Art of Whetting Your Own Appetite* is the ability to identify our desires. This art encourages us to really locate what we want. If we can name it, we can claim it, baby!

2. *The Womanly Art of Having Fun No Matter What* means that no matter the circumstances, we recognize and choose pleasure. Whether we're at the dry cleaners, at work, or changing diapers, we can find a way to have *fun*.

3. *The Womanly Art of Sensual Pleasure* locates women in this eternal truth: that each glorious inch of our body is ours to use for our own fulfillment. We explore and learn our body's capacity to experience pleasure, and make sure we always get ours. (All while using protection, of course!)

4. *The Womanly Art of Flirtation* is the act of a woman accessing her life force through her delight and joy in herself, in the presence of another. By doing so we create fun and turn-on in everyone around us.

5. *The Womanly Art of Owning Your Own Beauty* means making the decision, every minute of every day, that we are the hottest, most gorgeous things that ever lived.

6. *The Womanly Art of Partying with Your Inner Bitch* is the discipline of righteously channeling our anger as our biggest ally.

7. *The Womanly Art of Owning and Operating Men (or Women!)* is the ability to use our pleasure to navigate the vicissitudes of our relationships with grace and humor—all the while having our way.

8. *The Womanly Art of Inviting Abundance* is the art of harnessing the force of nature that is within us and using it to attract life's riches.

The Tools of the Womanly Arts

1. *Bragging and Upriding:* Brag to get off on yourself, feel your value, and take your listener higher too. Upride, or praise, someone who has bragged and make the experience for them—and you—twice as fun.

2. *Gratitude Lists:* A great exercise to reach for when you are feeling lack, disappointment, or like you just aren't getting yours. Unacknowledged good turns to constipation. Making a Gratitude List can ensure that you are celebrating the gold in your life.

3. *Desire Lists:* Tap into your personal magic and co-create your heart's desires with the Great Pussy in the Sky by writing a Desire List.

4. *Favorite Frames/Digestion:* A powerful way to process experiences is by framing (reporting to someone) the peak pleasure rides you took within those experiences.

5. *Spring Cleaning:* By doing this exercise, you dump the intense emotions on any topic so you can stay connected to your pleasure, which leads to inner guidance and knowing.

6. *Dance Breaks:* Anytime. Anywhere. Put on your favorite music and embody ecstatic movement to reenliven, refresh, or digest emotions and thoughts nonverbally. Dancing awakens and enlivens your being, flooding you with all kinds of feel-good hormones, which drench your cells in health.

7. *Womantra:* Break the habit of negative thinking by replacing unconscious messages with conscious, juicy, goddessly reframes that you have written for yourself. Examples include: "I am beautiful and fabulous and everything goes my way today!" "I am a ripe, dripping peach, just out of reach!" "I have the hottest pussy in [name your city]!"

8. *Self-Pleasure:* A woman's sensuality is her true source of power. Stay connected to all of you by self-pleasuring just for fun or when you require self-care before asking for a raise at work, or parenting at home, or preparing for a big date with a new guy or gal. Self-pleasuring does not necessarily mean giving yourself an orgasm. It might be that you just take a few pleasure-filled strokes of your pussy in order to make her feel good. The idea is to tap into your body's natural ability to wash and refresh your cells with the chemistry of pleasure. The greatest gift you can give yourself is to connect, on the regular, with your birthright of passion and ecstasy. I recommend a drop of lube as you stroke yourself to smooth the way for greater pleasure.

9. *Act of Anonymous Good:* Take your pleasure by taking someone higher. By doing anonymous acts of good, you start to feel good about yourself and the way you are showing up in the world, which adds to your radiance.

10. *Conjuring:* Conjuring is the manifestation of our desire, a living tribute to our power as women to attract. The act of conjuring means taking your pleasure from the yearning for whatever it is you desire.

11. *Defensive Dating:* This is the practice of dating a bunch of guys or gals at once, having a good time all around without putting all your eggs in one basket.

12. *Approval:* Make him a hero, or her a heroine. Show your enjoyment and appreciation for that special person in your life. A smile, a thank-you, a statement of gratitude goes a long way. Your approval must outweigh your demands.

13. *Training Cycle:* Three simple steps make up the Training Cycle.

> a) Show your partner that she/he is right.
> b) Give him/her a problem that he/she can solve.
> c) Acknowledge your partner.

14. *Pussify:* Make it beautiful. Get in there, take over, and glorify your closet, underwear drawer, office, or list of friends! Create space in your life for beauty. Keep only what makes you feel that way.

15. *Bitte et Chat:* Focus your attention on another. Think pleasant, delicious thoughts about your pussy, or the pussy or cock of the person you are focusing on. Direct your thoughts any way that turns you on. Notice how this simple thought creates a lot of fun and flirtation!

16. *Pleasure Diet:* A rigorous list of small to large pleasurable activities done to increase your light.

17. *Pleasure Basket:* A basket filled with something for all your senses. Include anything that makes your bedroom your playroom. A Sister Goddess lives her sensuality every day. Keep your Pleasure Basket fresh and fun.

18. *Sister Goddess Activism:* Change a woman's life today. We are all sisters on this planet. When you place your pleasure-filled attention on another woman in order to take her higher, that's activism!

19. *Flirt:* Flirt with the first person or thing that passes you. Flirtation is nothing more or less than enjoying yourself in the presence of another person.

20. *Shout "YES!":* No matter where you are, leap straight into the air and give a big "Yes!" when something you are in total disagreement with happens. It's a quick way of getting into agreement with and celebrating your life.

21. *Decorate Your Pussy:* Throw a few pretty stickers, tattoos, or body jewels on your hot bod and you will feel refreshed, revived, and resanctified.

22. *Gratitude:* Express your gratitude for someone you appreciate, right now.

23. *Flash Yourself:* Give yourself a pussy flash in the mirror and say, "This hot body is loved." It will change your chemistry to send a bit of love your own way.

24. *Go Panty-Free:* Do it on Friday, or any day of the week. Notice how you feel free. (And a bit naughty.)

25. *Give Yourself One Small Stroke of Pleasure:* Light a candle on your desk, buy yourself a flower, put on perfume . . . you get the idea. Every time you pleasure yourself, you set a pussy free somewhere in this world.

26. *Perfect and Elegant Womantra:* Repeat to yourself, "My timing is perfect and elegant. I am in exactly the right place at the right time." This ancient Sister Goddess Womantra re-creates your relationship with time so you can feel the pleasure of the moment and bend time to your will.

27. ***Wardrobe Change:*** Put on your tiara, boa, or garbage bag—or all three if necessary. Every woman feels best when her insides match her outsides. When you wear a crown, you will feel like a queen. A boa will remind you to flirt. And yes, a trash bag can shorten the amount of time you spend feeling like garbage.

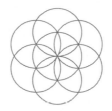

FURTHER
RESOURCES

There are so many wonderful resources out there that will expand, deepen, and broaden your understanding of the topics covered in this book. This list covers some of my favorites, but it is by no means exhaustive! Find your own, and share them with your friends—and with me, on the School of Womanly Arts Facebook page (see the next page).

Mama Gena's School of Womanly Arts

Come one, come all, through the doors of Mama Gena's School of Womanly Arts! The school is my masterpiece, my creation, my gift to you. Inside its doors you will find a deeper path toward everything you want most.

Entry is free. Simply visit our website, www.mamagenas.com, to begin your journey.

The site is chock-full of amazing information just waiting for you to scoop up and enjoy. Sign up for my newsletter if you want to hear from me and other radiant women on the same path you're on. Read up on our course offerings, and join the movement!

Community

SWA Facebook page: www.facebook.com/mamagena

Books by yours truly

Mama Gena's School of Womanly Arts: Using the Power of Pleasure to Have Your Way with the World

Mama Gena's Owner's and Operator's Guide to Men

Mama Gena's Marriage Manual: Stop Being a Good Wife, Start Being a Sister Goddess!

Books by other wonderful people

Woman: An Intimate Geography by Natalie Angier

The Story of V: A Natural History of Female Sexuality by Catherine Blackledge

Femalia by Joani Blank

Extended Massive Orgasm by Steve Bodansky, Ph.D., and Vera Bodansky, Ph.D.

The Yoni: Sacred Symbol of Female Creative Power by Rufus C. Camphausen

Slow Sex: The Art and Craft of the Female Orgasm by Nicole Daedone

Sacred Pleasure: Sex, Myth, and the Politics of the Body by Riane Eisler

The Book of the Courtesans: A Catalogue of Their Virtues by Susan Griffin

Cuffed, Tied, and Satisfied: A Kinky Guide to the Best Sex Ever by Jaiya

Sister Outsider by Audre Lorde (a great collection of essays; I particularly recommend "Uses of the Erotic: The Erotic as Power")

Cunt: A Declaration of Independence by Inga Muscio

Women's Bodies, Women's Wisdom: Creating Physical and Emotional Health and Healing by Christiane Northrup, M.D.

Seductress: Women Who Ravished the World and Their Lost Art of Love by Betsy Prioleau

The Game of Life and How to Play It by Florence Scovel Shinn

Women's Anatomy of Arousal and *Succulent SexCraft* by Sheri Winston

Recommended courses

Lafayette Morehouse – www.lafayettemorehouse.com

This is where I did my own sensual training. Brilliant content. Not for the faint of heart.

OneTaste – www.onetaste.us

OneTaste offers courses in Orgasmic Meditation (OM), man-woman dynamics, and communication all over the world.

Layla Martin – www.layla-martin.com

Layla publishes weekly videos about sex and teaches wonderful online classes for singles and couples.

Sheri Winston – www.intimateartscenter.com

Sheri is the real deal and knows more about pussy than anyone I have ever met.

Jaiya – www.missjaiya.com

Jaiya is "hands on, hands in," as she would say. Amazing, heartfelt, intuitive instruction.

Other resources

S Factor – www.sfactor.com

Created by my friend Sheila Kelley, S Factor is the best body movement for women that I have ever encountered. She taught me how to move this woman's body, and everything started to make a new kind of sense.

The Business of Being Born (2008) – www.thebusinessofbeing born.com

This powerful documentary by executive producer Ricki Lake and filmmaker Abby Epstein is a must-see for anyone considering having a baby.

Vulva Puppet

Can't wait to get your hands on a plush pussy like the one described on page 45? Believe me, I understand. There are many places you can find them on the Internet, but my favorite is: www.etsy.com/shop/WondrousVulvaPuppet.

OMGYES –www.omgyes.com

This is, by far, the greatest website for pussy education and training in existence. It was the brainchild of two friends who saw an unfulfilled need in understanding, articulating, and teaching people about what pussies like and how they work. They assembled a phenomenal team to guide users through video trainings and fingers-on experiences. They hit it right out of the park. One small stroke for pussy. One giant leap for womankind.

Ranier Wood – www.vulvere.com

Beautiful, reflective art from the artist who created the pussy drawing on page 92.

References

Engel, Pamela. "MAP: Divorce Rates around the World." *Business Insider,* May 25, 2014.

Hamilton, Brady E., et al. "Births: Final Data for 2014." *National Vital Statistics Reports* (National Center for Health Statistics) 64, no. 12 (2015).

Hanes, Stephanie. "Singles Nation: Why So Many Americans Are Unmarried." *Christian Science Monitor,* June 14, 2015.

Kantor, Jodi. "Harvard Business School Case Study: Gender Equity." *The New York Times,* September 7, 2013.

National Marriage Project. *The State of Our Unions.* 2012: The National Marriage Project, Charlottesville, VA.

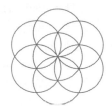

ACKNOWLEDGMENTS

There are so many amazing teachers, friends, lovers, family, co-conspirators, rebels, trailblazers, and overall badasses who have had a huge helping hand in the creation of this book. Not to mention the thousands upon thousands of women who blew open or barreled through so many doors that I never even knew existed, who made me possible and made this book possible. I am forever in your debt. To be able to live my unique truth is a gift I am cartwheelingly grateful for every single day.

Imagine *that*, Bubbe Rose and Grandma Regina, and all of my ancestresses before you. Because of *you*, I get to live my truth and live my gifts and make a great living in freedom. Thank you for risking all you risked in leaving your old world and coming to this new world and making me possible.

I want to give my unending gratitude and eternal love to my mama, Bebe Magness Weiss, and to my other mama, Miss Wilma Harris. I would not be the woman I am today without their magnificent love and the powerful, unstoppable ways I watched each of these women step up and say yes to life. My mama has been the Bubbe not only to her eight grandchildren, but also to thousands of women in the Mastery classroom, wiping their tears and sending them back into the game, revived and restored. Her deep, eternal love has been my lifeline. My Wilma, who always called me "Girlie," taught me through words and silence how to retain my dignity in a world of intolerance.

Thank you, Maggie Rose, the most amazing, smart, brilliant, beautiful, fun, and funny daughter on earth. You inspire me to be stronger and better than I could have ever been without you.

I am so overwhelmingly blessed to have Ruth Barron, my person, who supports me—and the SWA—with unimaginable love, fun, and seriously hot tracks. Ruth imagined herself into the role of Song Siren (DJ to the soul of woman), the very first time I taught Mastery. She has been by my side, steadfastly and magically creating the impossible-to-resist soundtrack of our lives, for every woman in Mastery, both inside and outside of the room. I would not be able to do the work I do, as well as I do it, without Ruth by my side. I am the most blessed woman on earth to have attracted such an incredible friend.

I thank my amazing editor, Kelly Notaras, who held such strong space as this book began to emerge her way into the world. What a blessed and beautiful collaboration—you held a spotlight on my soul with your passionate attention. I could not have asked for nor dreamed of better support.

I am so so grateful for my Hay House editor, Anne Barthel, who brought her gentle slash-and-burn to bear on whatever wasn't absolutely essential. She is like a spa treatment—everything gets refreshed, firmer, and tighter.

Thank you to Patty Gift, my friend and co-conspirator. I am so grateful that you lured me into the Hay House family.

Thank you, Reid Tracy and Louise Hay. What a joy to work with a passionate company that knows how to launch books.

Kris Carr. Sigh. In your graceful unicornly way, you have had my back and my front, top, bottom, and both sides throughout the creation of this book and its launch into the world.

Marie Forleo, I still remember the day I drove to your house in a holy terror when I realized what the title of this book had to be. You supported my vision then, now, and always. Thank you for your fierce friendship.

I am so grateful to Amanda Brooks, not just for the endless fashion inspiration and forcing me to spend way more on "investment pieces" than I ever thought possible, but for her endless love and support of me, and my work, for the past 20 years.

I am so unbelievably grateful to my team:

The glorious Donna Otmani, with whom I have worked and laughed with for more than 10 years. Your leadership and direction makes it all happen.

Nathan Patmor, who has woven in and out of my life for over a decade, always taking me, and my company, to our next level of growth and development. I love jumping off cliffs with you. You make soft landings.

I am so honored to work with Lauren Abrami and Hannah Williams. These two women are the portal through which every student enters the SWA. They are both beautiful, brilliant, impassioned, and filled with a fiery creativity that continues to inspire me, every day.

Rica Bryan for the unimaginable art form of mic running.

I want to thank Sarah Granby and Julie Nelson for creating such beautiful live events, managing runways with 1,000 women, and creating live stage magic with me.

Thank you, Susan Lee, for your incredible art direction and the most gorgeous book cover. Your amazing ability to take the not-yet-formed image in my head and place it beguilingly on the page is phenomenal.

Extraordinary gratitude to the artist Ranier Wood for her gorgeous pussy illustration included in this book.

Deep deep unending gratitude to Ayo, Mercedes, Bernadette, Omo, and all of my past and present event staff who bring it, lay it down, and burn it up with me each course weekend. This could not happen without you.

I am so grateful to the artist Jaq Belcher for creating the sacred geometry of the endsheets and allowing the book to call in its perfect audience.

The joy of working with the brilliant sexy photographer Liz Linder, both inside the Mastery classroom room and inside this book cover, cannot be underestimated. Thank you for meeting my exuberance with your own.

I am so grateful to have Osnat Yaski as my personal assistant / friend / support team. She has helped me keep all the balls in play for five glorious years.

Thank you, Colleen Maloney, for thousands of healthy, beautiful meals that nourish me and Maggie each week.

Deep gratitude to Becca Jones for managing our office so beautifully.

And to Carmen, my sister, my friend, my support, and the woman who keeps our home and office sparkling.

Special thanks to Dr. Anne Davin, who helped co-create the five phases of the Courtesan's Journey with me and contributed so much to the School of Womanly Arts.

I am so deeply indebted to have my steadfast pals Lydia Littlefield Danz, Joan Courtney Murray, and Kate O'Neill, who have been in my life for 40 years. To have the privilege of our lifelong friendship is something I am grateful for every single day.

I am so profoundly indebted to Nicole Daedone, Sheila Kelley, Betty Dodson, Jaiya, Barbara Stanny, Chris Northrup, Debbie Rosas, Kris Carr, Marie Forleo—the women who are barreling down the highway of setting pussies free and empowering men and women to heights heretofore unknown. Your work means so much to me. Thank you for showing up and speaking at Mastery.

And there simply are no words to express the gratitude I feel to each and every one of my students. I am grateful to the early adopters, the brave pioneers from the brownstone days, who took my class 20 years ago, when we were just a handful of women in my living room doing all kinds of crazy, amazing, outrageous things.

I am so overwhelmed with gratitude to the women who have done Mastery, and to the women who are currently in Mastery, where it still feels like we are as close and intimate as it did in my living room, still doing crazy, amazing, outrageous things. Thank you for your impossible courage in saying yes to a long-buried part of you that so wanted to breathe free and fly high.

I am so so so grateful to my Creation Course graduates. You took the deep dive with me. I know your insides and your outsides like I know my own soul. Thank you for your lust for going deep. Thank you for your insistence on excellence. Thank you for your courage and beauty.

I am grateful for my Virtual Pleasure Bootcampers from all over the country and the world. You kicked some serious butt. Now drop and give me a Holy Trinity!!

And to all the women who have been Big Sisters in the School of Womanly Arts, I am on bended knee before you. Thank you for holding space for women, for choosing to become mentors, for your incredible leadership, for forging new pathways for women as you make your way in the world.

And to the incredible astonishing unstoppable Team Pleasure, truly 8,000 nerve endings at your service. Thank you for making the impossible possible. Thank you for taking four white mice and making them four white horses. Thank you for the endless boxes of Kleenex, handfuls of rose petals, courtesan couches, and pink feathers. Thank you for your passionate attention.

Thank you Shonda Rhimes, Beyoncé, Tracy Chapman, Macy Gray, Lauryn Hill, Kate Bush, Barry Manilow, Alanis Morissette, Bruce Springsteen, Freddie Mercury, David Bowie, David Gray, The Who, Puccini, Låpsley, Mae West, Tina Turner, Sheryl Sandberg, Susan B. Anthony, Mary Oliver, Oprah, Maya Angelou, Judy Chicago, Sojourner Truth, Harriet Tubman, Alice Walker, Lena Dunham, Jennifer Lawrence, Lena Horne, Khia, Diane von Furstenberg, Mickalene Thomas, Lin-Manuel Miranda, Hillary Clinton, Elizabeth Gilbert, POTUS and Michelle Obama, Jane Goodall—the inspirational people whom I have not (yet) all met, but who keep the fire in my belly alive.

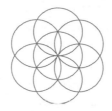

ABOUT THE AUTHOR

Regena Thomashauer (a.k.a. "Mama Gena") is a revolution: an icon, teacher, author, mother, and founder and CEO of the School of Womanly Arts. She believes that women are the greatest untapped natural resource on the planet, and she teaches them to turn on their innate feminine power to create a life they love.

The School for Womanly Arts began in Thomashauer's living room in 1998 and has since grown into a thriving global movement, with thousands of graduates around the world, more than 2,500 students annually, as well as tens of thousands of followers via her popular blog and online presence.

Thomashauer's approach stems from decades of research in the social, cultural, and economic history of women, including the ancient Goddess religion, which dominated 30 to 50 centuries of recorded history. She opens doors for women with her distinctive style, which is at once irreverent, unwavering, inspirational, and moving.

In addition to leading the School, Thomashauer has been featured widely as a leading expert in modern feminism.

She has authored three popular books published by Simon & Schuster: *Mama Gena's School of Womanly Arts: Using the Power of Pleasure to Have Your Way with the World* (2002), *Mama Gena's Owner's and Operator's Guide to Men* (2003) and *Mama Gena's Marriage Manual* (2004).

As a speaker, Thomashauer has been featured at TEDxFiDi-Women, the Wharton School of Business at the University of

Pennsylvania, the Young Presidents' Organization, Hillcrest Hospital, Cleveland Clinic, and the Health and Wellness Center by Doylestown Hospital, among others.

In the media, she has appeared as a frequent guest on NBC-TV's *Today* show, *Late Night with Conan O'Brien*, as well as *20/20*, *The Ricki Lake Show*, *The Rachael Ray Show*, *Lifetime Live*, *The Other Half*, and more.

Her programs have been profiled in esteemed publications including *The New York Times, Elle, Elle UK*, and *New York* magazine. Thomashauer's unique perspective has also been quoted in *Glamour, Newsweek, Marie Claire, Allure, Self, InStyle*, and *The Washington Post*.

Thomashauer graduated with a BA in Theater Arts from Mount Holyoke College before pursuing the reclamation of women's potential for the past 25 years. She lives and works in New York City, raising her daughter and working with a devoted team to run and grow the School of Womanly Arts.

Hay House Titles of Related Interest

YOU CAN HEAL YOUR LIFE, the movie, starring Louise Hay & Friends
(available as a 1-DVD program, an expanded 2-DVD set,
and an online streaming video)
Learn more at www.hayhouse.com/louise-movie

THE SHIFT, the movie,
starring Dr. Wayne W. Dyer
(available as a 1-DVD program, an expanded 2-DVD set,
and an online streaming video)
Learn more at www.hayhouse.com/the-shift-movie

*GODDESSES NEVER AGE: The Secret Prescription for Radiance,
Vitality, and Well-Being,* by Christiane Northrup, M.D.

*QUANTUM LOVE: Use Your Body's Atomic Energy
to Create the Relationship You Desire,* by Laura Berman, Ph.D.

*RADICAL SELF-LOVE: A Guide to Loving Yourself
and Living Your Dreams,* by Gala Darling

*WORTHY: Boost Your Self-Worth to Grow Your
Net Worth,* by Nancy Levin

All of the above are available at your local bookstore,
or may be ordered by contacting Hay House (see next page).

We hope you enjoyed this Hay House book. If you'd like to receive our online catalog featuring additional information on Hay House books and products, or if you'd like to find out more about the Hay Foundation, please contact:

Hay House, Inc., P.O. Box 5100, Carlsbad, CA 92018-5100
(760) 431-7695 or (800) 654-5126
(760) 431-6948 (fax) or (800) 650-5115 (fax)
www.hayhouse.com® • www.hayfoundation.org

Published and distributed in Australia by:
Hay House Australia Pty. Ltd., 18/36 Ralph St., Alexandria NSW 2015
Phone: 612-9669-4299 • *Fax:* 612-9669-4144 • www.hayhouse.com.au

Published and distributed in the United Kingdom by:
Hay House UK, Ltd., Astley House, 33 Notting Hill Gate, London W11 3JQ
Phone: 44-20-3675-2450 • *Fax:* 44-20-3675-2451 • www.hayhouse.co.uk

Published in India by: Hay House Publishers India,
Muskaan Complex, Plot No. 3, B-2, Vasant Kunj, New Delhi 110 070
Phone: 91-11-4176-1620 • *Fax:* 91-11-4176-1630 • www.hayhouse.co.in

Distributed in Canada by:
Raincoast Books, 2440 Viking Way, Richmond, B.C. V6V 1N2
Phone: 1-800-663-5714 • *Fax:* 1-800-565-3770 • www.raincoast.com

Access New Knowledge.
Anytime. Anywhere.

Learn and evolve at your own pace
with the world's leading experts.

www.hayhouseU.com

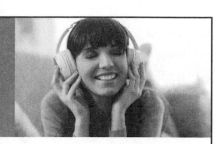

Hay House Podcasts
Bring Fresh, Free Inspiration Each Week!

Hay House proudly offers a selection of life-changing audio content via our most popular podcasts!

Hay House Meditations Podcast

Features your favorite Hay House authors guiding you through meditations designed to help you relax and rejuvenate. Take their words into your soul and cruise through the week!

Dr. Wayne W. Dyer Podcast

Discover the timeless wisdom of Dr. Wayne W. Dyer, world-renowned spiritual teacher and affectionately known as "the father of motivation." Each week brings some of the best selections from the 10-year span of Dr. Dyer's talk show on HayHouseRadio.com.

Hay House World Summit Podcast

Over 1 million people from 217 countries and territories participate in the massive online event known as the Hay House World Summit. This podcast offers weekly mini-lessons from World Summits past as a taste of what you can hear during the annual event, which occurs each May.

Hay House Radio Podcast

Listen to some of the best moments from HayHouseRadio.com, featuring expert authors such as Dr. Christiane Northrup, Anthony William, Caroline Myss, James Van Praagh, and Doreen Virtue discussing topics such as health, self-healing, motivation, spirituality, positive psychology, and personal development.

Hay House Live Podcast

Enjoy a selection of insightful and inspiring lectures from Hay House Live, an exciting event series that features Hay House authors and leading experts in the fields of alternative health, nutrition, intuitive medicine, success, and more! Feel the electricity of our authors engaging with a live audience, and get motivated to live your best life possible!

Find Hay House podcasts on iTunes, or visit
www.HayHouse.com/podcasts for more info.